100 WEIGHT LOSS TIPS

TABLE OF CONTENTS

 *INTRODUCTION

CHAPTER 1: SET REALISTIC GOALS

CHAPTER 2: TRACK YOUR PROGRESS

CHAPTER 3: DRINK MORE WATER

CHAPTER 4: AVOID SUGARY DRINKS

CHAPTER 5: INCLUDE PROTEIN IN EVERY MEAL

CHAPTER 6: EAT MORE FIBER-RICH FOODS

CHAPTER 7 : TAKE REGULAR WALKS

CHAPTER 8: FOCUS ON WHOLE FOODS

CHAPTER 9: AVOID PROCESSED FOODS

CHAPTER 10: PRACTICE PORTION CONTROL

CHAPTER 11: FOCUS ON GUT HEALTH

CHAPTER 12: INCORPORATE DAILY STRETCHING

CHAPTER 13: AVOID SKIPPING MEALS

CHAPTER 14: EXPLORE ANTI-INFLAMMATORY FOODS

CHAPTER 15: INCLUDE VEGETABLES IN EVERY MEAL

CHAPTER 16: PLAN YOUR MEALS

CHAPTER 17: AVOID EATING LATE AT NIGHT

CHAPTER 18: STAY CONSISTENT

CHAPTER 19: ADD EXERCISE TO YOUR ROUTINE

CHAPTER 20: CHOOSE LOW-CALORIE SNACKS

CHAPTER 21: AVOID EATING OUT OFTEN

CHAPTER 22: TRY A PLANT-BASED DIET FOR WEIGHT LOSS

CHAPTER 23: USE OLIVE OIL INSTEAD OF BUTTER

CHAPTER 24: REDUCE CARBOHYDRATE INTAKE

CHAPTER 25: EAT MORE PROTEIN-RICH SNACKS

CHAPTER 26: MEAL PREPIN ADVANCE

CHAPTER 27: TRY INTERMITTENT FASTING

CHAPTER 28: TRACK YOUR CALORIES

CHAPTER 29: DRINK GREEN TEA

CHAPTER 30: INCLUDE HEALTHY SNACKS IN YOUR DAY

CHAPTER 31: MAKE VEGETABLES A PART OF EVERY MEAL

CHAPTER 32: REDUCE SUGAR IN YOUR DIET

CHAPTER 33: GET ENOUGH SLEEP

CHAPTER 34: INCORPORATE HEALTHY FATS

CHAPTER 35: PRACTICE MINDFUL EATING

CHAPTER 36: REDUCE ALCOHOL CONSUMPTION

CHAPTER 37: PRACTICE SELF-DISCIPLINE

CHAPTER 38: PRACTICE REGULAR EXERCISE

CHAPTER 39: STAY HYDRATED

CHAPTER 40: KEEP A FOOD DIARY

CHAPTER 41: USE STANDING DESKS OR ACTIVE SITTING

CHAPTER 42: CONSUME PROTEIN WITH EVERY MEAL

CHAPTER 43: HOW TO USE FITNESS APPS TO STAY ON TRACK

CHAPTER 44: ROTATE YOUR WORKOUT ROUTINE

CHAPTER 45: LEARN TO COOK LOW-CALORIE RECIPES

CHAPTER 46: EAT BALANCED DIET

CHAPTER 47: INCLUDE FIBER-RICH

CHAPTER 48: JOIN A FITNESS CLASS OR GROUP

CHAPTER 49: USE HERBS AND SPICES FOR FLAVOR

CHAPTER 50: LEVERAGE STRESS MANAGEMENT TO AVOID STRESS EATING

CHAPTER 51: AVOID HIGH-CALORIE BEVERAGES

CHAPTER 52: CHOOSE WHOLE GRAINS OVER REFINED GRAINS

CHAPTER 53: LIMIT PROCESSED MEATS

CHAPTER 54: REPLACE SUGARY SNACKS WITH FRUIT

CHAPTER 55: AVOID HIGH-CALORIE SAUCES

CHAPTER 56: CHOOSE GRILLED OR BAKED FOODS

CHAPTER 57: LIMIT YOUR INTAKE OF REFINED SUGAR

CHAPTER 58: EAT MORE SOUP

CHAPTER 59: CONTROL YOUR HUNGER WITH HEALTHY SNACKS

CHAPTER 60:EAT HIGH-VOLUME, LOW-CALORIE FOODS

CHAPTER 61: TRY YOGA OR PILATES FOR FLEXIBILITY

CHAPTER 62: DRINK HERBAL TEAS

CHAPTER 63: MAKE YOUR OWN SNACKS

CHAPTER 64: LIMIT TAKEOUT AND FAST FOOD

CHAPTER 65: AVOID EXCESSIVE SALT

CHAPTER 66: GET SUPPORT FROM FRIENDS OR FAMILY

CHAPTER 67: USE FERMENTED FOODS TO BOOST IMMUNE FUNCTION

CHAPTER 68: OPT FOR DARK CHOCOLATE INSTEAD OF MILK CHOCOLATE

CHAPTER 69: MAKE HEALTHY SWAPS FOR COMFORT FOODS

CHAPTER 70: ADD MORE FIBER TO YOUR DIET

CHAPTER 71: KEEP YOUR STRESS UNDER CONTROL

CHAPTER 72: INCORPORATE STRENGTH TRAINING TO BUILD MUSCLE

CHAPTER 73: SKIP SUGARY CEREALS FOR BREAKFAST

CHAPTER 74: EAT MORE LOW-FAT DAIRY PRODUCTS

CHAPTER 75: INCLUDE HEALTHY SNACKS BETWEEN MEALS

CHAPTER 76: REPLACE SODA WITH SPARKLING WATER

CHAPTER 77: DRINK WATER BEFORE MEALS

CHAPTER 78: INCLUDE LEAN PROTEINS IN EVERY MEAL

CHAPTER 79: PLAN YOUR MEALS IN ADVANCE

CHAPTER 80: EAT SLOWLY AND MINDFULLY

CHAPTER 81: STAY CONSISTENT WITH EXERCISE

CHAPTER 82: DRINK GREEN SMOOTHIES FOR DETOX AND ENERGY

CHAPTER 83: INCORPORATE MORE FRUITS AND VEGETABLES

CHAPTER 84: CHOOSE THE RIGHT SUPPLEMENTS TO SUPPORT WEIGHT LOSS

CHAPTER 85: AVOID ARTIFICIAL SWEETENERS

CHAPTER 86: TRACK YOUR PROGRESS

CHAPTER 87: CREATE A SUPPORT SYSTEM

CHAPTER 88: EAT MORE WHOLE FOODS

CHAPTER 89: USE HEALTHY SUBSTITUTES FOR BAKING

CHAPTER 90: STAY POSITIVE THROUGHOUT YOUR JOURNEY

CHAPTER 91: AVOID FAD DIET

CHAPTER 92: FOCUS ON LONG-TERM HEALTH

CHAPTER 93: ENJOY YOUR WEIGHT LOSS JOURNEY

CHAPTER 94: INCLUDE AVOCADOS IN YOUR DIET

CHAPTER 95: SETTING REALISTIC EXPECTATIONS

CHAPTER 96: AVOID THE "ALL OR NOTHING" MINDSET

CHAPTER 97: INCORPORATE PHYSICAL ACTIVITY

CHAPTER 98: REWARD YOURSELF

CHAPTER 99: STAY COMMITTED THROUGH CHALLENGES

CHAPTER 100: MAINTAINING YOUR WEIGHT LOSS

***CONCLUSION**

INTRODUCTION

Achieving and maintaining a healthy weight is a journey that requires commitment, knowledge, and consistency. 100 Weight Loss Tips serves as a comprehensive guide to help you navigate this journey effectively. Whether you're just starting or seeking to refine your existing strategies, these practical tips cover every aspect of weight management, from nutrition and exercise to mindset and lifestyle changes.

This book emphasizes sustainable approaches rather than quick fixes. You'll discover how to set realistic goals, make healthier food choices, and incorporate physical activity seamlessly into your daily routine. With insights into mindful eating, meal planning, and staying motivated, you'll learn to build habits that promote long-term success.

Each tip is designed to be actionable and adaptable, ensuring that you can personalize them to fit your lifestyle. From choosing high-volume, low-calorie foods to limiting takeout, these strategies empower you to take control of your health. Additionally, the book addresses common challenges such as emotional eating, portion control, and staying active despite a busy schedule.

By following these tips, you can create a balanced lifestyle that not only helps you lose weight but also enhances your overall well-being. Let this guide be your companion on the path to a healthier, happier you.

CHAPTER 1: SET REALISTIC GOALS

1.1 UNDERSTANDING THE IMPORTANCE OF SETTING GOALS
Setting realistic goals is crucial for successful weight loss. Goals provide direction, motivation, and a clear roadmap for achieving your desired results. Unrealistic goals can lead to frustration and discouragement when progress is slower than expected. By setting attainable goals, you can maintain motivation, track your progress, and celebrate small successes along the way.

1.2 HOW TO SET SMART GOALS
To set realistic weight loss goals, apply the SMART criteria:

*SPECIFIC: Your goal should be clear and well-defined. For example, "I want to lose 10 pounds in 3 months."

*MEASURABLE: Make sure you can track your progress, such as losing 2 pounds per week.

*ACHIEVABLE: The goal should be challenging but not impossible. Losing 1-2 pounds per week is considered healthy and attainable.

*RELEVANT: Ensure the goal aligns with your overall health and wellness journey.

*TIME-BOUND: Set a specific timeframe to achieve the goal, such as 3 months.

1.3 BREAKING GOALS INTO SMALLER STEPS
Instead of focusing on one big goal, break it down into smaller, manageable steps. For example:

*SHORT-TERM GOALS: Losing 2 pounds this week, increasing daily water intake.

*MEDIUM-TERM GOALS: Exercising for 30 minutes a day, eating vegetables with every meal.

*LONG-TERM GOALS: Reaching your target weight and maintaining it for a specific period.

1.4 REVIEW AND ADJUST GOALS AS NECESSARY
Regularly assess your progress and be willing to adjust your goals if needed. Life circumstances can change, and your initial plan may need tweaking to remain realistic.

CHAPTER 2: TRACK YOUR PROGRESS

2.1 WHY TRACKING IS IMPORTANT
Tracking your progress helps you stay accountable and measure the effectiveness of your efforts. It allows you to identify patterns, celebrate milestones, and spot areas where you may need to improve. Tracking also provides motivation, as seeing tangible results can encourage you to keep going.

2.2 WAYS TO TRACK YOUR WEIGHT LOSS
There are several methods to track your progress:

*WEIGHT SCALE: Weigh yourself weekly, not daily, to avoid fluctuations due to water retention and other factors.

*MEASUREMENTS: Track your waist, hips, chest, and thigh measurements to monitor changes in body composition.

*FOOD LOG: Keep a daily food journal to record what you eat, portion sizes, and calorie intake.

*PHOTOS: Take progress pictures every month to visually track changes in your body.

*EXERCISE LOG: Keep a record of your workouts to monitor improvements in strength, endurance, and consistency.

2.3 USING TRACKING TOOLS AND APPS
Leverage technology to make tracking easier. Apps like MyFitnessPal and Lose It! can help you log your food intake, exercise, and even track your weight. These apps provide data analysis to help you stay on track.

CHAPTER 3: DRINK MORE WATER

3.1 THE ROLE OF WATER IN WEIGHT LOSS
Drinking water is one of the simplest and most effective weight loss tips. Water helps keep you hydrated, suppresses appetite, aids digestion, and boosts metabolism. Many

times, thirst is confused with hunger, leading to overeating. Staying hydrated can help prevent unnecessary calorie consumption.

3.2 HOW MUCH WATER SHOULD YOU DRINK?
A common recommendation is to drink at least 8 cups (64 ounces) of water a day. However, individual water needs vary depending on factors like body size, activity level, and climate. Some experts suggest drinking half your body weight in ounces. For example, if you weigh 150 pounds, aim for 75 ounces of water per day.

3.3 STRATEGIES TO DRINK MORE WATER

*CARRY A WATER BOTTLE: Keep a reusable bottle with you at all times to remind yourself to drink.

*SET REMINDERS: Use your phone or a water-tracking app to send reminders to drink throughout the day.

*ADD FLAVOR: If plain water feels boring, add a slice of lemon, cucumber, or mint to enhance the taste.

*DRINK BEFORE MEALS: Drinking a glass of water before meals can help curb your appetite and prevent overeating.

CHAPTER 4: AVOID SUGARY DRINKS

4.1 WHY SUGARY DRINKS HINDER WEIGHT LOSS
Sugary drinks like sodas, fruit juices, and energy drinks are high in empty calories, which provide little to no nutritional value. These beverages can quickly add hundreds of calories to your diet, contributing to weight gain. Moreover, sugary drinks spike your blood sugar, leading to energy crashes and cravings.

4.2 CALORIE CONTENT OF COMMON DRINKS

*A 12-ounce can of soda contains about 150 calories, all from sugar.

*A 16-ounce glass of fruit juice can have upwards of 200 calories and just as much sugar.

*Sweetened coffee or tea drinks can easily add 300-400 calories per serving.

4.3 ALTERNATIVES TO SUGARY DRINKS

*WATER: The best calorie-free option for hydration.

*SPARKLING WATER: A fizzy alternative without sugar or calories.

*UNSWEETENED TEA: Green tea, black tea, or herbal tea, without added sugar, provides flavor and hydration.

*COFFEE: Drink black coffee or coffee with minimal milk or unsweetened alternatives.

4.4 HOW TO QUIT SUGARY DRINKS

*START SMALL: If you're used to sugary drinks, cut back gradually to reduce cravings.

*READ LABELS: Check the sugar content of drinks to make informed decisions.

*REPLACE WITH HEALTHIER OPTIONS: Replace sugary drinks with healthier choices like water or unsweetened teas.

CHAPTER 5: INCLUDE PROTEIN IN EVERY MEAL

5.1 WHY PROTEIN IS ESSENTIAL FOR WEIGHT LOSS
Protein plays a crucial role in weight loss by promoting satiety, which helps you feel fuller longer. It also boosts metabolism and helps preserve lean muscle mass while you're losing fat. High-protein diets have been shown to increase calorie burn and reduce overall appetite.

5.2 BENEFITS OF PROTEIN FOR WEIGHT LOSS

*INCREASED METABOLISM: Protein requires more energy to digest than carbohydrates or fats, leading to more calories burned.

*PRESERVING MUSCLE MASS: When you lose weight, you often lose muscle along with fat. Protein helps prevent this.

*BETTER SATIETY: Protein-rich foods help you feel satisfied and less likely to overeat.

5.3 SOURCES OF PROTEIN
Include protein-rich foods in every meal, such as:

*ANIMAL SOURCES: Chicken, turkey, fish, lean beef, eggs, and dairy products.

*PLANT SOURCES: Lentils, beans, quinoa, tofu, tempeh, nuts, and seeds.

5.4 HOW TO INCORPORATE MORE PROTEIN INTO YOUR DIET

*ADD PROTEIN TO EVERY MEAL: Include a protein source with each breakfast, lunch, and dinner.

*SNACK ON PROTEIN: Opt for protein-packed snacks like Greek yogurt, nuts, or hard-boiled eggs.

*PROTEIN SMOOTHIES: Blend protein powder with fruits and vegetables for a nutritious snack or meal.

CHAPTER 6: EAT MORE FIBER-RICH FOODS

6.1 WHY FIBER IS IMPORTANT FOR WEIGHT LOSS
Fiber is a crucial component in a weight loss plan because it helps regulate digestion, maintain healthy blood sugar levels, and increase feelings of fullness. High-fiber foods take longer to digest, keeping you satisfied for longer periods and reducing overall calorie intake. Fiber also helps prevent constipation, supports gut health, and may lower the risk of chronic diseases.

6.2 TYPES OF FIBER
There are two main types of fiber:

*SOLUBLE FIBER: Dissolves in water to form a gel-like substance that helps control blood sugar levels and lowers cholesterol. Found in oats, beans, and fruits like apples and oranges.

*INSOLUBLE FIBER: Adds bulk to your stool, promoting regular bowel movements. Found in whole grains, vegetables, and wheat bran.

6.3 FIBER-RICH FOODS TO INCLUDE IN YOUR DIET

*LEGUMES: Lentils, beans, and chickpeas are high in fiber and protein, making them ideal for weight loss.

*VEGETABLES: Broccoli, spinach, kale, and carrots are rich in fiber and low in calories.

*FRUITS: Apples, pears, and berries are excellent sources of fiber.

*WHOLE GRAINS: Brown rice, quinoa, oats, and whole wheat bread should replace refined grains in your diet.

6.4 TIPS FOR INCREASING FIBER IN YOUR DIET

*Add a fiber supplement if necessary.

*Snack on fruits or vegetables like carrots or apples.

*Include legumes in soups, salads, and stews.

CHAPTER 7: TAKE REGULAR WALKS

7.1 THE BENEFITS OF WALKING FOR WEIGHT LOSS

Walking is one of the simplest and most effective forms of exercise. It requires no special equipment, can be done anywhere, and fits into even the busiest of schedules. Regular walking not only burns calories but also boosts your metabolism, making it a powerful tool for weight loss.

7.2 HOW WALKING AIDS WEIGHT LOSS

Walking helps you create a calorie deficit, which is essential for weight loss. A brisk 30-minute walk can burn between 150-200 calories, depending on your weight and pace.

Additionally, walking improves circulation, enhances cardiovascular health, and strengthens your muscles, all of which contribute to a healthier body.

7.3 INCORPORATING WALKING INTO YOUR ROUTINE

1. START SMALL: If you're new to walking, begin with short 10-15 minute sessions and gradually increase the duration.
2. SET GOALS: Aim for at least 10,000 steps per day. Use a pedometer or a fitness app to track your steps and stay motivated.
3. CHOOSE CONVENIENCE: Walk during your lunch break, take the stairs instead of the elevator, or park farther from your destination to add extra steps.

7.4 MAKING WALKING ENJOYABLE

1. EXPLORE NEW ROUTES: Keep your walks interesting by exploring different neighborhoods or parks.
2. WALK WITH A FRIEND: Walking with a companion can make the experience more enjoyable and help you stay consistent.
3. LISTEN TO MUSIC OR PODCASTS: Keep your mind engaged while walking by listening to your favorite tunes or educational podcasts.

7.5 COMBINING WALKING WITH OTHER HABITS

Walking can be paired with other healthy habits for even better results. For instance, take a walk after meals to aid digestion or use it as a form of active meditation to clear your mind. When combined with a balanced diet, regular walking can significantly accelerate your weight loss journey.

7.6 CONSISTENCY IS KEY

The key to benefiting from walking is consistency. Make it a daily habit, and over time, you'll notice improvements not just in your weight but in your overall physical and mental health. Walking is a low-impact exercise, making it suitable for people of all fitness levels, and it provides a sustainable way to stay active for life.

By taking regular walks, you're setting a strong foundation for long-term weight management and overall well-being.

CHAPTER 8: FOCUS ON WHOLE FOODS

8.1 WHAT ARE WHOLE FOODS?
Whole foods are unprocessed or minimally processed foods that are close to their natural state. Examples include fruits, vegetables, whole grains, lean proteins, and legumes. These foods are packed with essential nutrients and free from added sugars, unhealthy fats, and preservatives found in processed foods.

8.2 WHY WHOLE FOODS ARE BETTER FOR WEIGHT LOSS
Whole foods are nutrient-dense, meaning they provide a lot of essential vitamins, minerals, and fiber for fewer calories. They also tend to have lower amounts of unhealthy fats and added sugars, which can lead to weight gain.

8.3 HOW TO INCORPORATE MORE WHOLE FOODS INTO YOUR DIET

*Choose fresh produce over canned or processed versions.

*Replace refined grains (like white rice and white bread) with whole grains.

*Focus on lean meats, fish, eggs, and plant-based proteins instead of processed meats.

CHAPTER 9: AVOID PROCESSED FOODS

9.1 THE DANGER OF PROCESSED FOODS
Processed foods are often high in unhealthy fats, sugars, and sodium, all of which contribute to weight gain and other health issues. These foods are designed for convenience, but they offer little nutritional value and can lead to overeating.

9.2 HOW PROCESSED FOODS AFFECT WEIGHT LOSS

*EMPTY CALORIES: Processed foods often contain added sugars and fats that contribute to weight gain without providing essential nutrients.

*LOW SATIETY: These foods don't fill you up, causing you to eat more and still feel hungry.

*INCREASED CRAVINGS: Many processed foods, especially those high in sugar, can trigger cravings for more unhealthy snacks.

9.3 HOW TO AVOID PROCESSED FOODS

*Stick to fresh, whole foods whenever possible.

*Avoid packaged snacks like chips, cookies, and sugary drinks.

*Cook meals at home to control the ingredients and avoid hidden sugars and unhealthy fats.

CHAPTER 10: PRACTICE PORTION CONTROL

10.1 WHY PORTION CONTROL MATTERS
Even healthy foods can contribute to weight gain if you consume them in large portions. Portion control helps prevent overeating by teaching you how to gauge appropriate serving sizes and eat mindfully.

10.2 TIPS FOR EFFECTIVE PORTION CONTROL

*Use smaller dishes and bowls.

*Read food labels to understand the recommended serving sizes.

*Practice mindful eating by paying attention to your hunger and fullness cues.

10.3 COMMON PORTION CONTROL MISTAKES

*Eating directly from packages or large containers.

*Overestimating portion sizes, especially at restaurants.

*Eating out of boredom or stress, rather than true hunger.

CHAPTER 11: FOCUS ON GUT HEALTH

11.1 UNDERSTANDING GUT HEALTH

Your digestive system plays a crucial role in your overall health, influencing everything from immunity to weight loss. Maintaining a healthy gut can help regulate metabolism, reduce inflammation, and improve nutrient absorption, all of which are key factors in weight management. The gut microbiome—the community of bacteria living in your intestines—can be positively or negatively affected by your diet, lifestyle, and stress levels.

11.2 HOW GUT HEALTH AFFECTS WEIGHT LOSS

A healthy gut microbiome can help balance your hormones, including those that regulate hunger and fat storage. An imbalance in gut bacteria has been linked to weight gain, poor digestion, and inflammation. Therefore, focusing on gut health is essential for long-term weight loss success.

11.3 FOODS THAT PROMOTE GUT HEALTH

*FERMENTED FOODS: These foods are rich in probiotics, which can help improve gut health by increasing beneficial bacteria. Examples include yogurt, kefir, sauerkraut, and kimchi.

*FIBER-RICH FOODS: High-fiber foods such as fruits, vegetables, legumes, and whole grains feed the healthy bacteria in your gut, promoting digestion and a healthy microbiome.

*PREBIOTICS: These are foods that feed the beneficial bacteria, such as garlic, onions, asparagus, and bananas.

11.4 TIPS TO IMPROVE GUT HEALTH

*Add a variety of fiber and fermented foods to your diet.

*Avoid excessive sugar and processed foods, as they can harm the gut microbiome.

*Stay hydrated to support digestion.

*Manage stress, as chronic stress can disrupt gut health.

CHAPTER 12: INCORPORATE DAILY STRETCHING

12.1 The Importance of Stretching
Stretching is not just for flexibility; it plays an important role in overall health, especially when it comes to weight loss. Incorporating daily stretching routines helps improve circulation, reduce muscle stiffness, enhance flexibility, and prevent injuries. Regular stretching also helps in lowering stress levels, which is crucial for weight management.

12.2 HOW STRETCHING CONTRIBUTES TO WEIGHT LOSS
While stretching itself doesn't directly burn many calories, it can aid in weight loss by:

*Increasing mobility, allowing for better performance in more intense workouts like cardio or strength training.

*Reducing stress, which can prevent stress-induced overeating.

*Improving posture, leading to more energy throughout the day, and reducing back pain that may prevent physical activity.

12.3 TYPES OF STRETCHING TO INCLUDE

*STATIC STRETCHING: This involves holding a stretch for 20-30 seconds and is useful for improving flexibility and muscle recovery after workouts.

*DYNAMIC STRETCHING: This involves moving parts of your body and gradually increasing reach, speed of movement, or both. It's ideal before workouts to prepare your muscles for activity.

*YOGA: Incorporating yoga into your daily routine can help improve flexibility, strength, and relaxation, supporting both physical health and mental well-being.

12.4 TIPS FOR DAILY STRETCHING

*Set aside time each day for a stretching routine, even if it's just 10-15 minutes.

*Focus on full-body stretches that target the legs, arms, back, and neck.

*Don't rush—stretch to the point of mild discomfort, but not pain.

*Practice breathing deeply during stretches to promote relaxation.

CHAPTER 13: AVOID SKIPPING MEALS

13.1 WHY SKIPPING MEALS IS A BAD IDEA
Skipping meals can lead to overeating later in the day, as hunger hormones increase and you may feel ravenous. It also slows down metabolism, making it harder to lose weight.

13.2 THE IMPORTANCE OF REGULAR MEALS
Eating at regular intervals ensures steady energy levels, prevents blood sugar spikes, and helps manage hunger throughout the day.

13.3 STRATEGIES TO AVOID SKIPPING MEALS

*Prepare meals in advance for busy days.

*Keep healthy snacks on hand to avoid temptation.

*Set regular meal times and stick to them.

CHAPTER 14: EXPLORE ANTI-INFLAMMATORY FOODS

14.1 UNDERSTANDING INFLAMMATION AND WEIGHT LOSS
Chronic inflammation is a common condition linked to various health problems, including obesity, heart disease, and diabetes. It can slow down metabolism, making weight loss more difficult. Inflammation can be caused by a poor diet, stress, and environmental toxins. By incorporating anti-inflammatory foods into your diet, you can reduce inflammation and help support your weight loss efforts.

14.2 BENEFITS OF ANTI-INFLAMMATORY FOODS
*Anti-inflammatory foods work by fighting the inflammation in the body, reducing insulin resistance, and promoting a healthier metabolism.

*These foods can also help regulate hormones associated with hunger, which can support weight loss.

*Additionally, they provide your body with essential vitamins, minerals, and antioxidants that improve overall health.

14.3 BEST ANTI-INFLAMMATORY FOODS

*FATTY FISH: Salmon, mackerel, and sardines are rich in omega-3 fatty acids, which have powerful anti-inflammatory effects.

*BERRIES: Blueberries, strawberries, and blackberries are high in antioxidants called flavonoids that help reduce inflammation.

*LEAFY GREENS: Vegetables like spinach, kale, and collard greens are packed with vitamins and minerals that reduce inflammation.

*NUTS AND SEEDS: Walnuts, almonds, chia seeds, and flaxseeds are great sources of omega-3s and fiber that help reduce inflammation.

*TURMERIC AND GINGER: Both of these spices contain compounds that have anti-inflammatory properties and can help reduce overall inflammation in the body.

14.4 TIPS FOR ADDING ANTI-INFLAMMATORY FOODS TO YOUR DIET

*Make a habit of including fatty fish in your meals at least twice a week.

*Snack on berries or add them to your smoothies and yogurt.

*Include dark leafy greens in salads, soups, and stir-fries.

*Use turmeric and ginger in your cooking or in warm drinks like tea.

*Experiment with anti-inflammatory herbs and spices to add flavor to your meals.

CHAPTER 15: INCLUDE VEGETABLES IN EVERY MEAL

15.1 WHY VEGETABLES ARE IMPORTANT FOR WEIGHT LOSS

Vegetables are low in calories and high in fiber, making them perfect for weight loss. They are also packed with essential vitamins, minerals, and antioxidants that support overall health and metabolism.

15.2 TYPES OF VEGETABLES TO INCLUDE

*LEAFY GREENS: Spinach, kale, arugula, and collard greens are some of the healthiest vegetables, packed with vitamins A, C, K, and minerals like iron and calcium. They are low in calories and high in fiber, making them perfect for weight loss.

*CRUCIFEROUS VEGETABLES: Broccoli, cauliflower, Brussels sprouts, and cabbage are high in fiber, vitamins, and minerals. They also contain compounds that support detoxification and may reduce the risk of certain cancers.

*ROOT VEGETABLES: Carrots, sweet potatoes, and beets are rich in nutrients like beta-carotene, potassium, and fiber. They provide a healthy source of carbohydrates and are perfect for energy-boosting meals.

*ALLIUM VEGETABLES: Onions, garlic, leeks, and shallots are not only flavorful but also offer health benefits like improved immunity and heart health. They are also low in calories but provide a lot of flavor, making them ideal for various dishes.

*PEPPERS: Bell peppers (red, yellow, green) are rich in vitamin C and antioxidants. They are crunchy, low-calorie, and versatile for a variety of dishes.

15.3 HOW TO INCORPORATE MORE VEGETABLES INTO YOUR DIET

*START YOUR DAY WITH VEGETABLES: Add spinach or kale to your morning smoothie or omelette for a nutrient boost.

*INCLUDE VEGETABLES IN SNACKS: Snack on raw veggies like carrot sticks, cucumber slices, or bell pepper strips paired with hummus or a yogurt dip.

*USE VEGETABLES AS A BASE: Instead of relying on pasta or rice, use cauliflower rice or zucchini noodles. You can also blend vegetables into soups or stews for extra flavor and nutrition.

*MAKE VEGETABLES THE STAR: Fill half of your plate with vegetables at every meal. Make them the main part of the meal by pairing them with lean proteins or healthy fats.

*ADD VEGETABLES TO SMOOTHIES: For an extra nutritional boost, blend vegetables like spinach, kale, or carrots into your smoothies along with your fruits. This adds fiber and vitamins without altering the taste too much.

15.4 BENEFITS OF EATING MORE VEGETABLES

*WEIGHT MANAGEMENT: Due to their high fiber content, vegetables help with satiety, which can prevent overeating and aid in weight loss.

*NUTRIENT DENSITY: Vegetables are packed with essential vitamins and minerals that support overall health, including immunity, digestion, and energy levels.

*IMPROVED DIGESTION: The fiber in vegetables promotes healthy digestion and regular bowel movements, preventing constipation.

*LOWER DISEASE RISK: Regular consumption of vegetables has been linked to a reduced risk of chronic diseases such as heart disease, type 2 diabetes, and certain cancers.

15.5 SIMPLE WAYS TO COOK VEGETABLES

*ROASTING: Roasting vegetables like carrots, broccoli, or Brussels sprouts in the oven with a drizzle of olive oil and your favorite herbs can bring out their natural sweetness and flavor.

*STEAMING: Steaming preserves the nutrients in vegetables like broccoli, spinach, and green beans while keeping them tender and flavorful.

*STIR-FRYING: Stir-fry vegetables with lean proteins like chicken or tofu for a quick, healthy meal. Use a small amount of olive oil or coconut oil for cooking.

*GRILLING: Grilling vegetables like zucchini, peppers, and asparagus adds a smoky flavor and makes them more appetizing.

15.6 STRATEGIES TO MAKE EATING VEGETABLES A HABIT

*PLAN AHEAD: Include vegetables in your meal planning. Having pre-cut veggies in the fridge makes it easier to add them to your meals.

*GET CREATIVE WITH COOKING: Experiment with new vegetable recipes or try different cooking methods like roasting or grilling.

*MAKE VEGETABLES FUN: For kids or picky eaters, make vegetables more enjoyable by serving them with dips, mixing them into pasta dishes, or blending them into smoothies.

*COOK IN BATCHES: Prepare large quantities of vegetable-based soups or stews and store them in the fridge for quick and easy meals throughout the week.

15.7 FINAL THOUGHTS

Including a variety of vegetables in every meal not only helps with weight management but also contributes to better overall health. With their low calorie content, high fiber, and rich nutrient profile, vegetables are an essential part of any healthy diet. By getting creative and making vegetables the centerpiece of your meals, you can enjoy their benefits while keeping your meals delicious and satisfying.

*LEAFY GREENS: Spinach, kale, and arugula are nutrient-dense and low in calories.

CHAPTER 16: PLAN YOUR MEALS

16.1 WHY MEAL PLANNING MATTERS

Meal planning is an essential step toward successful weight loss. By planning your meals, you avoid the temptation of unhealthy snacks and convenience foods. It also helps you stick to a calorie-controlled diet and ensures you're consuming a balanced variety of foods. Meal planning saves time and money by eliminating impulse buying and frequent takeout meals.

16.2 HOW TO PLAN YOUR MEALS

*SET A WEEKLY MENU: Take 30 minutes every week to plan your meals. Create a shopping list based on your menu, focusing on whole foods like lean proteins, vegetables, fruits, and whole grains.

*BATCH COOKING: Prepare large quantities of meals at once, such as soups, stews, or casseroles. Store them in the fridge or freezer for later use.

*USE PORTION CONTROL: Pre-portion your meals into containers, so you know exactly how much to eat. This can help you avoid overeating.

*CHOOSE BALANCED MEALS: Each meal should contain protein, healthy fats, fiber, and some carbs. This helps stabilize blood sugar and keeps you full longer.

16.3 BENEFITS OF MEAL PLANNING

*PREVENTS OVEREATING: With planned meals, you avoid the temptation to eat unhealthy snacks or overeat at mealtimes.

*SAVES TIME: With meals prepared ahead of time, you won't have to rush around cooking during busy days.

ENCOURAGES HEALTHY CHOICES: Planning meals ahead lets you choose healthier ingredients and portion sizes.

CHAPTER 17: AVOID EATING LATE AT NIGHT
17.1 THE IMPACT OF NIGHT-TIME EATING ON WEIGHT LOSS

Eating late at night can sabotage your weight loss efforts. Late-night eating disrupts your circadian rhythm, making it harder for your body to metabolize food efficiently. It often leads to overeating, as you might consume more calories than necessary when tired or stressed.

17.2 WHY LATE-NIGHT EATING IS PROBLEMATIC

*SLOWER METABOLISM AT NIGHT: Your metabolism naturally slows down in the evening, which means food consumed late is more likely to be stored as fat.

*DISRUPTED SLEEP: Eating large meals late at night can interfere with your sleep quality, leaving you tired and hungry the next day.

*MINDLESS EATING: Late-night snacks are often consumed out of boredom or habit rather than hunger, leading to unnecessary calorie consumption.

17.3 STRATEGIES TO AVOID LATE-NIGHT EATING

*SET A CUT-OFF TIME: Try to stop eating 2-3 hours before bedtime.

*EAT BALANCED MEALS: Consuming a nutritious dinner that includes protein and fiber can help you stay full and prevent late-night cravings.

*FIND HEALTHY ALTERNATIVES: If you must have a snack, opt for healthy options like a handful of nuts or a piece of fruit.

CHAPTER 18: STAY CONSISTENT

18.1 WHY CONSISTENCY IS KEY
Consistency is crucial for weight loss. Results take time, and fluctuating between unhealthy habits and strict diets can hinder progress. Staying consistent with healthy habits—whether it's eating balanced meals or exercising regularly—ensures long-term success.

18.2 HOW TO STAY CONSISTENT WITH YOUR GOALS

*SET REALISTIC EXPECTATIONS: Understand that weight loss is a gradual process. Set achievable goals to avoid frustration.

*CREATE HEALTHY HABITS: Build habits like meal prepping, exercising, and drinking water into your routine. These habits make it easier to stick to your goals.

*STAY MOTIVATED: Keep track of your progress with apps or a fitness journal. Celebrate small victories to stay motivated.

18.3 BENEFITS OF CONSISTENCY

*FASTER RESULTS: The more consistent you are with your healthy habits, the quicker you'll see results.

*IMPROVED CONFIDENCE: Sticking to a routine can help you feel empowered and more confident about your weight loss journey.

CHAPTER 19: ADD EXERCISE TO YOUR ROUTINE

19.1 THE IMPORTANCE OF EXERCISE FOR WEIGHT LOSS

Exercise not only burns calories but also builds muscle, boosts metabolism, and improves overall health. It's a vital part of any weight loss plan because it accelerates fat burning and enhances the effects of a balanced diet.

19.2 TYPES OF EXERCISE FOR WEIGHT LOSS

*CARDIOVASCULAR EXERCISE: Activities like running, cycling, or swimming increase your heart rate and burn calories. Aim for at least 150 minutes of moderate-intensity cardio per week.

*STRENGTH TRAINING: Lifting weights or using resistance bands helps build lean muscle mass, which burns more calories at rest.

*HIGH-INTENSITY INTERVAL TRAINING (HIIT): Short bursts of intense exercise followed by rest periods. HIIT can burn more calories in less time and is effective for fat loss.

19.3 HOW TO MAKE EXERCISE A HABIT

*START SLOW: Begin with moderate-intensity activities and gradually increase the intensity as your fitness improves.

*FIND ACTIVITIES YOU ENJOY: Exercise doesn't have to be a chore. Find activities you enjoy, like dancing, hiking, or playing sports.

*SET A ROUTINE: Make exercise part of your daily schedule. Whether it's in the morning or after work, consistency is key.

CHAPTER 20: CHOOSE LOW-CALORIE SNACKS

20.1 WHY SNACKING MATTERS
Snacking can either support or sabotage your weight loss goals. Choosing low-calorie snacks that are high in nutrients can help curb hunger and provide energy without excessive calories.

20.2 TYPES OF LOW-CALORIE SNACKS

*FRESH FRUITS: Apples, berries, and oranges are low-calorie, high-fiber snacks that satisfy sweet cravings.

*VEGETABLES WITH HUMMUS: Carrots, cucumber, and bell peppers paired with hummus are nutrient-packed and filling.

*GREEK YOGURT: Unsweetened Greek yogurt is rich in protein and can be topped with a small handful of nuts or berries.

*NUTS: While nuts are calorie-dense, a small portion can provide healthy fats and protein that curb hunger.

20.3 HOW TO CHOOSE THE RIGHT SNACKS

*READ LABELS: Always check for added sugars or unhealthy fats in packaged snacks.

*PRE-PORTION SNACKS: To avoid overeating, pre-portion your snacks into small containers.

*INCLUDE PROTEIN AND FIBER: Choose snacks that combine protein and fiber to keep you fuller for longer.

CHAPTER 21: AVOID EATING OUT OFTEN

21.1 THE CHALLENGE OF EATING OUT

Restaurant meals are often high in calories, fats, and sodium. Portion sizes are larger, and it's difficult to control ingredients when dining out. Eating out frequently can derail weight loss progress and lead to unhealthy choices.

21.2 HOW TO AVOID EATING OUT TOO MUCH

*COOK AT HOME: Preparing meals at home allows you to control ingredients, portions, and cooking methods.

*PLAN MEALS IN ADVANCE: If you know you'll be busy, plan quick, healthy meals for those days.

*FIND HEALTHIER RESTAURANT OPTIONS: If you must eat out, choose grilled, steamed, or baked dishes instead of fried foods.

21.3 BENEFITS OF COOKING AT HOME

*BETTER PORTION CONTROL: When you cook, you can control portion sizes and the ingredients you use.

*COST-EFFECTIVE: Cooking at home is often less expensive than eating out, especially when you buy in bulk.

CHAPTER 22: TRY A PLANT-BASED DIET FOR WEIGHT LOSS

A plant-based diet is not just a trend, but a powerful tool for weight loss and overall well-being. By focusing on whole, unprocessed plant foods, you can achieve sustainable weight loss while also reaping the numerous health benefits that come with this lifestyle. Here's how incorporating more plant-based foods into your diet can help you shed those extra pounds and improve your overall health.

22.1 UNDERSTANDING A PLANT-BASED DIET

A plant-based diet emphasizes the consumption of foods derived from plants, including vegetables, fruits, grains, nuts, seeds, and legumes. Unlike veganism, which excludes all animal products, a plant-based diet doesn't necessarily exclude everything; it simply prioritizes plant-derived foods while minimizing or eliminating animal-based foods.

This diet is rich in fiber, antioxidants, vitamins, and minerals, which not only support weight loss but also boost your immune system, improve digestion, and lower the risk of chronic diseases like heart disease, diabetes, and cancer. The fiber from plants helps you feel fuller longer, which can prevent overeating and snacking between meals.

22.2 HOW A PLANT-BASED DIET AFFECTS WEIGHT LOSS

The key to weight loss with a plant-based diet is reducing calorie intake while maintaining a high nutritional value. Here's how it works:

*LOWER IN CALORIES: Most plant-based foods are naturally low in calories, meaning you can eat larger portions without consuming excess calories. For example, a salad with vegetables, legumes, and avocado provides much fewer calories than a meal high in animal fats and processed foods.

*INCREASED FIBER INTAKE: Fiber plays a critical role in weight loss by making you feel full for longer periods. It also helps with digestion and can prevent constipation, a common issue in many weight loss plans.

*REDUCED INTAKE OF UNHEALTHY FATS: Plant-based diets typically exclude saturated fats found in animal products. Reducing saturated fat intake while increasing healthy fats from plant sources like avocados, nuts, and seeds can help reduce body fat over time.

*BOOST METABOLISM: Many plant foods, such as leafy greens, are packed with nutrients that help boost metabolism. For instance, spicy foods like chili peppers contain capsaicin, which has been shown to increase metabolism and promote fat burning.

22.3 COMMON PLANT-BASED FOODS TO INCLUDE IN YOUR DIET

To begin your plant-based journey, it's essential to know which foods to incorporate into your meals. Here are some key plant-based foods to include:

*VEGETABLES: Leafy greens like spinach, kale, and Swiss chard are nutrient-dense and low in calories. Other vegetables like broccoli, cauliflower, and carrots are also excellent choices.

*FRUITS: Berries, apples, bananas, and citrus fruits are packed with vitamins and antioxidants. They're low in calories, high in fiber, and perfect for satisfying your sweet tooth.

*LEGUMES: Beans, lentils, and chickpeas are high in protein and fiber, making them ideal for keeping you full and satisfied.

*WHOLE GRAINS: Brown rice, quinoa, oats, and whole wheat are great sources of fiber and can provide energy without causing spikes in blood sugar.

*NUTS AND SEEDS: Almonds, walnuts, chia seeds, and flaxseeds are excellent sources of healthy fats and protein.

*HEALTHY FATS: Avocados, olive oil, and coconut oil provide healthy fats that support brain function and help keep you satiated.

22.4 CREATING BALANCED MEALS

When transitioning to a plant-based diet, it's important to create balanced meals to ensure you're getting all the necessary nutrients. Each meal should contain:

*PROTEIN: Include plant-based protein sources like lentils, chickpeas, tofu, and edamame to maintain muscle mass and aid in recovery.

*HEALTHY FATS: Include a source of healthy fats, such as avocado or nuts, to support heart health and provide lasting energy.

*CARBOHYDRATES: Whole grains, sweet potatoes, and fruits provide complex carbohydrates, which give you the energy you need without spiking your blood sugar.

*FIBER: Vegetables, fruits, and whole grains provide fiber that promotes digestive health and helps regulate hunger.

22.5 TIPS FOR SUCCESS ON A PLANT-BASED DIET

*PLAN YOUR MEALS: Meal planning is essential when transitioning to a plant-based diet to avoid nutrient deficiencies and overeating. Make sure to include a variety of vegetables, grains, legumes, and healthy fats in your meals.

*BE MINDFUL OF PROTEIN: While plant-based protein sources are abundant, it's important to make sure you're consuming enough to meet your body's needs, especially if you're active. Include a variety of plant-based protein sources in your meals to ensure you're getting all the essential amino acids.

*AVOID PROCESSED PLANT-BASED FOODS: While there are many plant-based alternatives available, such as vegan cheese and fake meats, these can often be highly processed and contain added sugars and unhealthy fats. Stick to whole, minimally processed foods for the best results.

*STAY HYDRATED: Drinking plenty of water throughout the day helps with digestion and can keep you from feeling hungry when you're actually just thirsty.

*LISTEN TO YOUR BODY: Pay attention to how your body responds to plant-based foods. If you experience digestive discomfort, try different foods or adjust your intake of fiber to see what works best for you.

22.6 CONCLUSION

Adopting a plant-based diet for weight loss can be both effective and sustainable when done correctly. By focusing on whole, nutrient-dense foods, you can reduce calorie intake, increase fiber, and boost metabolism, all of which contribute to healthy weight loss. With the right planning and commitment, a plant-based diet can not only help you achieve your weight loss goals but also improve your overall health and well-being.

CHAPTER 23: USE OLIVE OIL INSTEAD OF BUTTER

23.1 INTRODUCTION
Switching from butter to olive oil is a simple yet impactful change you can make in your diet. Olive oil is not only a great source of healthy fats but also provides essential nutrients that butter lacks. If you are looking to lose weight and improve your overall health, this small change can make a big difference.

23.2 HOW TO USE OLIVE OIL IN YOUR COOKING

*SAUTEING AND STIR-FRYING: Olive oil is perfect for cooking at medium heat.

*SALAD DRESSINGS: Make homemade vinaigrette with olive oil, vinegar, and your favorite herbs.

*DRIZZLING ON VEGETABLES: Use olive oil to drizzle over roasted or steamed vegetables for extra flavor.

23.3 HEALTH BENEFITS OF OLIVE OIL
Olive oil is rich in monounsaturated fats, which are known to lower bad cholesterol (LDL) and raise good cholesterol (HDL). This can reduce your risk of heart disease and stroke. Additionally, olive oil contains powerful antioxidants like vitamin E, which help protect cells from damage caused by free radicals. Studies have also shown that olive oil has anti-inflammatory properties, which can benefit people with conditions like arthritis. Furthermore, it has been linked to improved blood sugar control and a reduced risk of developing type 2 diabetes.

23.4 HOW TO INCORPORATE OLIVE OIL INTO YOUR DIET
Olive oil can be used in various ways to replace butter in your cooking. Use it for sautéing vegetables or proteins, drizzling over salads, or as a base for marinades and dressings. You can even use olive oil in baking recipes where butter is traditionally used. Choose extra virgin olive oil for its higher antioxidant content and minimal processing. Be mindful of portion sizes, as olive oil is still calorie-dense.

CHAPTER 24: REDUCE CARBOHYDRATE INTAKE

24.1 INTRODUCTION
Reducing your carbohydrate intake is a proven way to lose weight effectively. While carbs are an important energy source, too many can lead to weight gain, especially refined carbohydrates that spike blood sugar levels and increase fat storage.

24.2 TYPES OF CARBOHYDRATES
Carbohydrates can be divided into two categories: simple and complex. Simple carbs, found in foods like white bread, pastries, and sugary snacks, are quickly digested, leading to insulin spikes and fat accumulation. Complex carbs, found in whole grains, vegetables, and legumes, are digested slowly, keeping blood sugar levels stable and helping with weight management.

24.3 HOW TO REDUCE CARBOHYDRATE INTAKE
To reduce carbs, focus on eliminating refined sugars and white flour-based products. Replace them with whole grains like quinoa, brown rice, oats, and barley. Incorporate more fiber-rich vegetables like leafy greens, broccoli, and cauliflower into your meals. Avoid sugary drinks and instead opt for water or herbal teas. By cutting back on high-glycemic foods, you'll help your body burn fat for fuel instead of relying on glucose from carbs.

CHAPTER 25: EAT MORE PROTEIN-RICH SNACKS

25.1 INTRODUCTION
Protein is a key nutrient in any weight loss plan. It helps build and repair muscle, boosts metabolism, and keeps you feeling fuller for longer. Replacing sugary or carb-heavy snacks with protein-rich options can significantly reduce your calorie intake and prevent overeating.

25.2 BENEFITS OF PROTEIN-RICH SNACKS
When you consume protein, it triggers the release of hormones that promote satiety, reducing hunger and cravings. Protein also increases thermogenesis, which is the process of burning calories to digest food. This can aid in fat loss while maintaining lean muscle mass. Eating protein-rich snacks throughout the day ensures you don't reach for unhealthy options when hunger strikes.

25.3 EXAMPLES OF PROTEIN-RICH SNACKS
Some great protein-packed snacks include Greek yogurt, cottage cheese, boiled eggs, almonds, lean turkey slices, and protein bars or shakes. Plant-based protein sources like

chickpeas, tofu, and edamame also provide excellent options. Preparing these snacks in advance ensures you always have healthy choices available, even when you're on the go.

CHAPTER 26: MEAL PREP IN ADVANCE

26.1 INTRODUCTION

Meal prepping is a strategy that can save time, reduce stress, and help you make healthier food choices throughout the week. By planning and preparing your meals ahead of time, you're more likely to stick to your diet and avoid making impulsive, unhealthy food choices.

26.2 BENEFITS OF MEAL PREPPING

Meal prepping allows you to control portion sizes and ensures that you have nutritious meals available when you're hungry. It eliminates the temptation to eat fast food or processed snacks, which are often calorie-dense and low in nutrients. Prepping meals in advance also saves time, allowing you to focus on other aspects of your day instead of scrambling for food.

26.3 HOW TO MEAL PREP FOR SUCCESS

Start by planning your meals for the week. Choose balanced recipes that include lean proteins, whole grains, and plenty of vegetables. Cook in bulk and divide your meals into individual servings. Store them in airtight containers for easy grab-and-go options. Consider using a slow cooker or instant pot for convenience. Don't forget to prep snacks, like chopped veggies or fruit, to keep you on track throughout the day.

CHAPTER 27: TRY INTERMITTENT FASTING

27.1 INTRODUCTION

Intermittent fasting (IF) has become a popular method for weight loss. It involves cycling between periods of eating and fasting, which may help reduce calorie intake and improve metabolic health.

27.2 BENEFITS OF INTERMITTENT FASTING

IF helps regulate insulin levels and promotes fat burning, especially abdominal fat. It also improves cell repair processes and may reduce the risk of chronic diseases like heart disease and diabetes. Some research suggests that IF can increase lifespan and improve brain function.

27.3 HOW TO TRY INTERMITTENT FASTING

There are several ways to practice intermittent fasting. The most common method is the 16/8 approach, where you fast for 16 hours and eat during an 8-hour window. You can also try the 5:2 method, which involves eating normally for five days and restricting calories to around 500-600 on two non-consecutive days. Start slowly, allowing your body time to adjust, and remember to stay hydrated during fasting periods.

CHAPTER 28: TRACK YOUR CALORIES

28.1 INTRODUCTION

Tracking your calories is one of the most effective ways to ensure you are in a calorie deficit, which is essential for weight loss. By keeping track of what you eat, you can identify areas where you may be overeating and make more mindful food choices.

28.2 HOW TO TRACK YOUR CALORIES

There are several ways to track your calories. You can use food tracking apps like MyFitnessPal or Lose It!, or you can keep a written food journal. Record everything you eat and drink, including portion sizes. This will help you understand your calorie intake and adjust your diet accordingly. Remember to include snacks and condiments, as they can add up.

28.3 TIPS FOR SUCCESSFUL TRACKING

Be honest with yourself and track everything, even if it's just a small snack. Learn to estimate portion sizes or use a food scale to be more accurate. Over time, tracking your calories can become second nature, and you will have a better understanding of your eating habits.

CHAPTER 29: DRINK GREEN TEA

29.1 INTRODUCTION

Green tea is a popular beverage known for its many health benefits, including its potential to aid in weight loss. It contains compounds like catechins and caffeine that can boost metabolism and increase fat burning.

29.2 HEALTH BENEFITS OF GREEN TEA

The catechins in green tea are antioxidants that can increase fat oxidation, especially during exercise. Studies suggest that drinking green tea regularly can help reduce belly fat and improve overall body composition. Additionally, green tea has been linked to improved heart health, better brain function, and reduced risk of certain cancers.

29.3 HOW TO INCORPORATE GREEN TEA INTO YOUR ROUTINE

To reap the benefits of green tea, aim for 2-3 cups per day. Avoid adding sugar or artificial sweeteners, as this can counteract the health benefits. You can enjoy green tea hot or cold and try experimenting with flavors like lemon or ginger for added variety.

CHAPTER 30: INCLUDE HEALTHY SNACKS IN YOUR DAY

30.1 INTRODUCTION

Healthy snacks can play a crucial role in maintaining energy levels and curbing hunger throughout the day. Choosing nutrient-dense snacks can prevent overeating during meals and keep you on track with your weight loss goals.

30.2 BENEFITS OF HEALTHY SNACKS

Healthy snacks help regulate blood sugar levels and prevent energy crashes. They also keep your metabolism active and prevent the binge eating that can result from extreme hunger. Incorporating balanced snacks with protein, fiber, and healthy fats can help manage hunger and cravings.

30.3 HEALTHY SNACK IDEAS

Good options include raw vegetables with hummus, a handful of almonds, apple slices with peanut butter, or Greek yogurt with berries. Focus on snacks that are nutrient-dense and provide a combination of protein, fiber, and healthy fats to keep you satisfied. Avoid processed snacks that are high in sugar and unhealthy fats.

CHAPTER 31: MAKE VEGETABLES A PART OF EVERY MEAL

31.1 INTRODUCTION
Including vegetables in every meal is a simple yet powerful way to enhance your diet. Vegetables are packed with essential vitamins, minerals, fiber, and antioxidants, which can help improve digestion, boost immunity, and support overall health. Adding them to every meal ensures you meet your daily nutritional needs while promoting a healthy weight.

31.2 HEALTH BENEFITS OF VEGETABLES
Vegetables are low in calories and high in nutrients, making them ideal for weight management. Their high fiber content aids digestion, prevents constipation, and helps control blood sugar levels. Vegetables like spinach, kale, and broccoli are rich in antioxidants that reduce inflammation and protect cells from oxidative stress. They also provide essential vitamins like vitamin A, C, and K, which support skin health, immunity, and bone health.

31.3 HOW TO INCLUDE MORE VEGETABLES
To make vegetables a part of every meal, start by adding leafy greens to salads, smoothies, or wraps. You can also sauté or roast vegetables like carrots, zucchini, and bell peppers as a side dish. For breakfast, try incorporating spinach or kale into an omelet or adding vegetables to your morning smoothie. Experiment with new vegetable recipes to make your meals more exciting and colorful.

CHAPTER 32: REDUCE SUGAR IN YOUR DIET

32.1 INTRODUCTION
Reducing your sugar intake is a crucial step in improving your health. High sugar consumption is linked to obesity, diabetes, heart disease, and other chronic conditions. By cutting back on added sugars, you can improve your energy levels, reduce cravings, and maintain a healthier weight.

32.2 THE DANGERS OF EXCESS SUGAR
Excess sugar, especially in processed foods and sugary drinks, contributes to weight gain by increasing insulin levels, which promotes fat storage. Sugar also causes spikes in blood glucose levels, leading to crashes that trigger cravings for more sugar.

Consuming too much sugar can increase your risk of developing metabolic disorders like type 2 diabetes and cardiovascular disease.

32.3 HOW TO REDUCE SUGAR INTAKE

Start by reading food labels and avoiding products with added sugars, such as sodas, candy, and baked goods. Replace sugary snacks with fresh fruits like berries or apples, which provide natural sugars along with fiber and antioxidants. If you drink coffee or tea, try reducing the amount of sugar or switching to stevia or other natural sweeteners. Gradually cut back on sugar to help your taste buds adjust.

CHAPTER 33: GET ENOUGH SLEEP

33.1 INTRODUCTION

Sleep is one of the most important factors in maintaining a healthy weight and overall well-being. Lack of sleep can disrupt hormone levels, increase hunger, and affect metabolism. Prioritizing quality sleep is essential for regulating appetite, boosting energy, and improving overall health.

33.2 THE LINK BETWEEN SLEEP AND WEIGHT LOSS

Lack of sleep can interfere with your weight loss goals by increasing hunger and cravings, especially for high-calorie foods. Sleep deprivation also affects your metabolism and can lead to fat accumulation.

33.3 HOW SLEEP AFFECTS HORMONES

*LEPTIN AND GHRELIN: Sleep deprivation lowers leptin (the hormone that signals fullness) and increases ghrelin (the hormone that signals hunger), making you more likely to overeat.

*CORTISOL: Lack of sleep increases cortisol, a stress hormone that can promote fat storage, particularly around the belly.

33.4 TIPS FOR IMPROVING SLEEP

Aim for 7-9 hours of sleep each night. Create a relaxing bedtime routine, such as reading or practicing deep breathing exercises, to signal your body that it's time to wind down. Avoid caffeine and electronic devices at least an hour before bed, as they can interfere with sleep. Make sure your sleep environment is comfortable, dark, and quiet for better rest.

CHAPTER 37: PRACTICE SELF-DISCIPLINE

37.1 THE ROLE OF SELF-DISCIPLINE IN WEIGHT LOSS

Self-discipline is the cornerstone of any successful weight loss journey. It helps you stay committed to your goals, make healthier choices, and resist temptations that could derail your progress. Developing self-discipline ensures you remain consistent even when motivation wanes.

37.2 UNDERSTANDING SELF-DISCIPLINE

Self-discipline involves the ability to control your impulses and stay focused on long-term benefits rather than immediate gratification. In the context of weight loss, it means choosing nutritious meals over junk food, exercising regularly, and avoiding unhealthy habits.

37.3 STRATEGIES TO BUILD SELF-DISCIPLINE

1. SET CLEAR GOALS: Define your weight loss objectives and break them into smaller, achievable targets. Having a clear vision makes it easier to stay disciplined.
2. CREATE A ROUTINE: Establishing a daily schedule for meals, exercise, and sleep helps you form healthy habits that become second nature over time.
3. ANTICIPATE CHALLENGES: Identify situations where you're likely to face temptations, such as social gatherings or stressful days, and plan how to handle them.

37.4 OVERCOMING TEMPTATIONS

1. AVOID TRIGGERS: Keep unhealthy snacks out of sight and stock your kitchen with nutritious options.
2. PRACTICE MINDFUL EATING: Focus on your meals, savoring each bite, and recognize when you're full to avoid overeating.
3. USE POSITIVE REINFORCEMENT: Reward yourself for staying disciplined, such as buying new workout gear or enjoying a non-food-related treat.

37.5 STAYING ACCOUNTABLE

Accountability is a powerful motivator. Share your goals with a friend, join a support group, or use a fitness app to track your progress. Knowing that others are aware of your journey can reinforce your self-discipline.

37.6 LEARNING FROM SETBACKS

Setbacks are inevitable, but they don't define your journey. Use them as learning opportunities to understand your triggers and develop stronger coping mechanisms. Remember, self-discipline isn't about being perfect; it's about consistently making better choices.

37.7 THE LONG-TERM BENEFITS OF SELF-DISCIPLINE

Practicing self-discipline not only helps you achieve your weight loss goals but also instills habits that promote overall well-being. It empowers you to take control of your health, boosts your confidence, and fosters a sense of accomplishment.

By embracing self-discipline, you equip yourself with the mental strength needed to overcome challenges and sustain a healthy lifestyle for years to come.

CHAPTER 38: PRACTICE REGULAR EXERCISE

38.1 Introduction

Regular physical activity is essential for maintaining a healthy weight, improving cardiovascular health, and boosting mood. Incorporating exercise into your daily routine helps you burn calories, build muscle, and stay fit, contributing to long-term health benefits.

38.2 Benefits of Regular Exercise

Exercise promotes fat loss, improves muscle tone, and enhances metabolism. It also reduces the risk of chronic diseases like heart disease, diabetes, and obesity. Additionally, physical activity releases endorphins, which can help reduce stress, anxiety, and depression.

38.3 How to Incorporate Exercise into Your Routine

Aim for at least 150 minutes of moderate-intensity exercise or 75 minutes of vigorous exercise each week. Activities like walking, jogging, cycling, swimming, and strength training are all effective for improving health. Choose exercises you enjoy to stay motivated and make physical activity a regular part of your life.

CHAPTER 39: STAY HYDRATED

39.1 INTRODUCTION
Hydration is vital for maintaining overall health and supporting numerous bodily functions, including digestion, metabolism, and cognitive performance. Water makes up a significant portion of your body and is essential for every cell, tissue, and organ to function optimally.

39.2 THE IMPORTANCE OF HYDRATION
Water is crucial for regulating body temperature, removing waste through urine, and supporting the transportation of nutrients and oxygen to cells. Staying hydrated also aids in maintaining joint health, skin hydration, and digestive health. Dehydration can lead to fatigue, confusion, and even more severe health issues like kidney stones or urinary tract infections.

39.3 HOW TO STAY HYDRATED
Aim to drink at least 8 cups (2 liters) of water daily, though individual needs may vary based on age, activity level, and climate. In addition to drinking water, consume hydrating foods like watermelon, cucumbers, and soups. Limit sugary drinks, as they can contribute to dehydration. Carry a water bottle with you throughout the day to remind yourself to stay hydrated.

CHAPTER 40: KEEP A FOOD DIARY

40.1 INTRODUCTION
A food diary is a powerful tool for tracking your eating habits, understanding your nutritional intake, and identifying areas for improvement. By keeping a detailed record of everything you eat and drink, you can make more informed choices and stay accountable to your health goals.

40.2 THE BENEFITS OF A FOOD DIARY
A food diary can help you identify patterns in your eating habits, such as emotional eating or consuming too many unhealthy snacks. It also allows you to spot any nutritional deficiencies and make adjustments to improve your overall diet. Additionally,

tracking your food intake can be motivating, as you see your progress and achievements over time.

40.3 HOW TO KEEP A FOOD DIARY
Write down everything you eat and drink, including portion sizes, the time of day, and how you felt while eating. You can use a physical notebook or digital apps to make the process more efficient. Review your diary regularly to assess areas for improvement and set new health goals.

CHAPTER 41: USE STANDING DESKS OR ACTIVE SITTING

41.1 THE BENEFITS OF STANDING DESKS
Sedentary behavior is one of the major contributors to weight gain and poor health. Using standing desks or adopting active sitting techniques during your workday can help counteract the negative effects of prolonged sitting. Standing encourages more movement, improves posture, and helps boost calorie expenditure. It's a simple yet effective strategy to incorporate physical activity into your daily routine without requiring extra time for a workout.

41.2 HOW STANDING DESKS HELP WITH WEIGHT LOSS

*INCREASED CALORIE BURN: Standing burns more calories than sitting. Research shows that standing for an hour can burn up to 50% more calories than sitting.

*IMPROVED POSTURE: Standing helps align the spine and reduces the strain on your back, which can prevent discomfort and improve overall health.

*ENHANCED PRODUCTIVITY: Many people find that standing increases their focus and energy, allowing them to be more productive throughout the day.

41.3 ACTIVE SITTING AND ALTERNATIVES

*ERGONOMIC CHAIRS: If standing for long periods is not feasible, using an ergonomic chair or active sitting chair can help. These chairs promote better posture and engage core muscles while seated.

*BALANCE BALLS: Sitting on a balance ball engages your core and helps strengthen your muscles while maintaining good posture.

*FOOTRESTS: Using a footrest under your desk can encourage more active sitting, as it allows you to shift your weight and engage different muscle groups.

41.4 TIPS FOR IMPLEMENTING ACTIVE SITTING

*START SLOW: Gradually increase the amount of time you spend standing throughout the day. Start with 15-minute intervals and build up to longer periods.

*ALTERNATE POSITIONS: Mix standing with sitting on an ergonomic chair or balance ball to prevent fatigue and strain.

*TAKE BREAKS: Make it a habit to take short walking breaks every hour to stretch your legs and keep your blood circulation flowing.

CHAPTER 42: CONSUME PROTEIN WITH EVERY MEAL

42.1 INTRODUCTION
Protein is an essential macronutrient that plays a key role in muscle growth, repair, immune function, and hormone regulation. Including protein in every meal helps support these bodily functions and keeps you feeling full longer.

42.2 THE ROLE OF PROTEIN
Protein helps build and repair tissues, enzymes, and hormones in the body. It also aids in keeping muscles strong and maintaining healthy skin, hair, and nails. Including protein-rich foods in your meals helps curb hunger and reduce cravings, making it easier to manage your weight.

42.3 HOW TO INCLUDE MORE PROTEIN
Incorporate protein-rich foods such as lean meats, fish, eggs, dairy, legumes, and tofu into each meal. Consider adding protein powder to smoothies or snacks for an easy boost. By ensuring you have a good source of protein with every meal, you'll support muscle recovery and stay satisfied between meals.

CHAPTER 43: HOW TO USE FITNESS APPS TO STAY ON TRACK

Staying consistent with your fitness goals can be challenging, but fitness apps provide a helpful and accessible way to track progress, set goals, and maintain motivation. In this chapter, we'll explore how to use fitness apps effectively to stay on track with your weight loss and fitness journey.

43.1 UNDERSTANDING THE BENEFITS OF FITNESS APPS

Fitness apps offer a wide range of benefits that can make tracking and achieving fitness goals easier. Some of the key benefits include:

*CONVENIENCE: Fitness apps allow you to track your progress at any time and from anywhere, making them ideal for busy lifestyles.

*MOTIVATION: Many fitness apps offer features like goal setting, reminders, and progress tracking that help keep you motivated.

*CUSTOMIZATION: Fitness apps can be tailored to your specific needs, whether you're focusing on weight loss, strength training, or endurance.

*COMMUNITY SUPPORT: Many apps have social features that allow you to connect with friends or other users for extra accountability.

43.2 CHOOSING THE RIGHT FITNESS APP

There are many fitness apps available, each catering to different needs. When choosing the right app for your weight loss and fitness goals, consider the following:

*GOAL-SPECIFIC FEATURES: Look for apps that focus on your specific goals, such as weight loss, strength training, or flexibility.

*USER EXPERIENCE: Choose apps with a clean and intuitive interface that makes it easy to track your workouts, meals, and progress.

*INTEGRATIONS: Some apps integrate with wearable devices like fitness trackers or smartwatches, offering even more detailed insights into your activity levels.

*REVIEWS AND RECOMMENDATIONS: Check user reviews and seek recommendations to find apps with a proven track record of helping users achieve their goals.

43.3 HOW TO TRACK YOUR WORKOUTS

Once you've chosen your app, it's time to start using it to track your workouts. Here are some ways to stay consistent with your fitness tracking:

*LOG EVERY WORKOUT: Make sure to log every workout session, whether it's cardio, strength training, or a combination. Most apps allow you to input the type of exercise, duration, intensity, and even the number of sets and reps for strength training.

*MONITOR INTENSITY AND DURATION: Many fitness apps provide data on the intensity of your workouts, including heart rate or calories burned. Use this information to adjust the intensity and duration of your workouts over time.

*SET WEEKLY GOALS: Set weekly workout goals based on time, frequency, or intensity. This helps create a consistent routine and keeps you accountable.

*REVIEW YOUR PROGRESS: Regularly review your progress within the app. This allows you to see improvements over time and adjust your goals as necessary.

43.4 USE APP FEATURES TO TRACK CALORIES AND DIET

In addition to tracking workouts, many fitness apps also have nutrition-tracking features. Here's how you can use these features to stay on track with your weight loss goals:

*TRACK YOUR CALORIES: Most fitness apps allow you to log meals and snacks. Entering your meals helps you track the calories you're consuming, which is crucial for weight loss.

*SET DAILY CALORIE GOALS: Many apps allow you to set calorie targets based on your weight loss goals. Be sure to track your food intake carefully to meet these targets.

*MONITOR MACRONUTRIENTS: Many apps also allow you to track macronutrients (protein, carbohydrates, and fats). This can help ensure you're consuming the right balance of nutrients to support your weight loss and fitness goals.

*ADD FOOD SCANNING FEATURES: Many apps include barcode scanning features, making it easier to input the nutritional information for packaged foods.

43.5 TRACKING YOUR SLEEP AND RECOVERY

Rest and recovery are important aspects of any fitness program. Some apps track your sleep patterns, which can help you understand how well you're recovering from workouts. Here's how to track recovery effectively:

*TRACK SLEEP QUALITY: Use the sleep-tracking features to monitor how much sleep you're getting and its quality. Aim for 7–9 hours of sleep to optimize recovery and maintain energy levels.

*MONITOR HEART RATE VARIABILITY (HRV): Some fitness apps track your HRV, which can indicate how well your body is recovering. Low HRV may suggest overtraining or lack of recovery.

*ADJUST YOUR ROUTINE: If your app indicates poor sleep or low recovery, consider adjusting your workout routine to allow more rest.

43.6 STAY MOTIVATED WITH APP FEATURES

Fitness apps offer several features that can help you stay motivated throughout your journey:

*REMINDERS AND NOTIFICATIONS: Set reminders to work out, drink water, or log meals to keep yourself on track.

*GAMIFICATION AND REWARDS: Some apps offer rewards, badges, or milestones for achieving goals, adding an element of fun and competition.

*JOIN CHALLENGES: Participate in app-hosted challenges or create your own to stay engaged and motivated.

*TRACK STREAKS: Many apps track your streaks (consecutive days of logging meals or workouts), which can serve as extra motivation to stay consistent.

43.7 CONNECT WITH A SUPPORT NETWORK

Accountability is key when it comes to achieving weight loss and fitness goals. Fitness apps often include social features that allow you to:

*CONNECT WITH FRIENDS: Add friends within the app for mutual support and motivation. Share your progress and encourage each other.

*JOIN ONLINE COMMUNITIES: Participate in online groups or forums within the app to discuss fitness goals, share tips, and get advice from others.

*TRACK SHARED GOALS: Some apps allow users to share specific goals with others, creating a sense of community and mutual accountability.

43.8 CONCLUSION

Fitness apps can be powerful tools to help you stay on track with your weight loss and fitness goals. By choosing the right app, tracking your workouts and diet, using app features to monitor sleep and recovery, and staying motivated with reminders and support, you can achieve long-term success. Embrace the technology available and make it work for you in your pursuit of a healthier, more active lifestyle.

CHAPTER 44: ROTATE YOUR WORKOUT ROUTINE

44.1 THE IMPORTANCE OF WORKOUT VARIETY
Performing the same workout routine day in and day out can lead to plateaus in your fitness progress and can even increase the risk of injury. Rotating your workout routine keeps your muscles challenged, promotes balanced muscle development, and prevents boredom. Variety in workouts also helps target different aspects of fitness, such as strength, endurance, flexibility, and cardiovascular health.

44.2 BENEFITS OF ROTATING YOUR WORKOUT ROUTINE

*PREVENTS PLATEAUS: The body adapts to exercise over time. Changing up your routine ensures that your muscles continue to grow and adapt, leading to ongoing progress.

*REDUCES RISK OF INJURY: Repeating the same movements can increase the risk of overuse injuries. By alternating your workouts, you give different muscle groups time to recover.

*BOOSTS MOTIVATION: Trying new activities or exercises keeps things fresh and fun, increasing the likelihood that you'll stay consistent with your fitness routine.

44.3 HOW TO ROTATE YOUR WORKOUTS

*ALTERNATE BETWEEN CARDIO AND STRENGTH: Incorporate cardio-focused days (running, cycling, swimming) with strength training days (weightlifting, bodyweight exercises).

*TRY DIFFERENT FITNESS MODALITIES: Experiment with different types of exercise, such as yoga, Pilates, HIIT, kickboxing, or dance to work different muscle groups and improve your fitness level.

*FOCUS ON FULL-BODY WORKOUTS: Rotate between exercises that target different muscle groups (upper body, lower body, core) to ensure balanced development.

44.4 TIPS FOR CHANGING UP YOUR ROUTINE

*PLAN YOUR WEEK: Schedule specific workout types for each day, such as Monday for strength training, Wednesday for cardio, and Friday for flexibility.

*TRACK YOUR PROGRESS: Keep a workout journal to track what exercises you've done and how much weight or repetitions you've achieved.

*STAY OPEN TO NEW CHALLENGES: Occasionally try a new activity outside of your usual routine (e.g., rock climbing, a fitness class, or a new sport) to keep things exciting.

CHAPTER 45: LEARN TO COOK LOW-CALORIE RECIPES

45.1 THE POWER OF HOME-COOKED MEALS
Cooking at home allows you to control the ingredients, portions, and preparation methods, giving you the ability to create healthy meals tailored to your nutritional needs. By learning to cook low-calorie recipes, you can create satisfying dishes that support your weight loss goals without sacrificing flavor.

45.2 BENEFITS OF LOW-CALORIE RECIPES

*PORTION CONTROL: When you prepare meals at home, you can control portion sizes, helping to prevent overeating.

*REDUCED USE OF UNHEALTHY INGREDIENTS: Homemade meals typically have less added sugar, salt, and unhealthy fats compared to restaurant or packaged foods.

*NUTRIENT-DENSE Ingredients: Low-calorie recipes often include fresh vegetables, lean proteins, and whole grains, which are nutrient-dense and help with satiety.

45.3 HEALTHY LOW-CALORIE MEAL IDEAS

*BREAKFAST: A vegetable-packed omelet with egg whites, spinach, and mushrooms, served with a side of fruit.

*LUNCH: Grilled chicken salad with mixed greens, cherry tomatoes, cucumbers, and a light vinaigrette dressing.

*DINNER: Baked salmon with roasted vegetables (e.g., zucchini, broccoli, carrots), served with quinoa or brown rice.

*SNACKS: Veggies with hummus or a small bowl of Greek yogurt with fresh berries.

45.4 TIPS FOR COOKING LOW-CALORIE MEALS

*USE HEALTHY COOKING METHODS: Opt for grilling, baking, steaming, or sautéing instead of frying to reduce added calories from oils and fats.

*EXPERIMENT WITH HERBS AND SPICES: Use fresh herbs, spices, and citrus zest to enhance the flavor of your dishes without adding extra calories.

*REPLACE HIGH-CALORIE INGREDIENTS: Swap creamy dressings with balsamic vinegar or low-fat yogurt, or replace white pasta with zucchini noodles or spaghetti squash.

*BATCH COOKING: Prepare large batches of low-calorie meals and freeze portions for easy, healthy meals throughout the week.

CHAPTER 46: EAT A BALANCED DIET

46.1 INTRODUCTION
A balanced diet consists of a variety of foods that provide the necessary nutrients your body needs to function properly. Eating a variety of foods ensures you get an adequate intake of vitamins, minerals, protein, and healthy fats.

46.2 COMPONENTS OF A BALANCED DIET
A balanced diet includes fruits, vegetables, whole grains, lean proteins, and healthy fats. Each food group plays a vital role in maintaining health, from boosting immunity to supporting muscle function and digestion. A balanced diet also supports weight management and reduces the risk of chronic diseases like heart disease and diabetes.

46.3 HOW TO ACHIEVE A BALANCED DIET
Aim to fill half your plate with vegetables and fruits, one-quarter with lean protein, and one-quarter with whole grains. Include healthy fats from sources like avocados, nuts, and olive oil. Limit processed foods and added sugars, and focus on eating a wide range of foods to ensure you get all the necessary nutrients.

CHAPTER 47: INCLUDE FIBER-RICH FOODS

47.1 INTRODUCTION
Fiber is an essential part of a healthy diet, promoting digestive health, weight management, and heart health. Foods rich in fiber help you feel full longer and regulate blood sugar levels.

47.2 THE BENEFITS OF FIBER
Fiber aids in digestion by adding bulk to stool and preventing constipation. It also supports a healthy gut microbiome and lowers cholesterol levels. Consuming adequate fiber is associated with a lower risk of heart disease, type 2 diabetes, and certain cancers.

47.3 HOW TO INCLUDE MORE FIBER
Include fiber-rich foods like fruits, vegetables, legumes, whole grains, and nuts in your diet. Aim for at least 25-30 grams of fiber per day. Start by adding fiber to each meal, such as incorporating beans into salads or adding oats to smoothies.

CHAPTER 48: JOIN A FITNESS CLASS OR GROUP

48.1 THE BENEFITS OF GROUP FITNESS

Joining a fitness class or group offers numerous advantages that can significantly enhance your weight loss journey. Group workouts provide structure, accountability, and a sense of community, which can boost your motivation and make exercising more enjoyable.

1. MOTIVATION THROUGH GROUP ENERGY: Exercising with others creates a shared energy that keeps you motivated. Seeing others push through challenges can inspire you to give your best effort.
2. ACCESS TO EXPERT GUIDANCE: Many fitness classes are led by professional trainers who can guide you through proper techniques and create balanced workout routines.

48.2 TYPES OF FITNESS CLASSES AND GROUPS

There's a wide range of fitness classes and groups available to suit different preferences and fitness levels.
1. CARDIO CLASSES: Examples include Zumba, spinning, or aerobics, designed to get your heart rate up and burn calories.
2. STRENGTH TRAINING GROUPS: These focus on building muscle and improving strength through exercises like weightlifting or resistance training.
3. YOGA AND PILATES: Ideal for improving flexibility, balance, and mental well-being while still contributing to weight loss.
4. OUTDOOR GROUPS: Running clubs, hiking groups, or cycling teams offer fitness activities in a refreshing outdoor setting.

48.3 SOCIAL SUPPORT AND ACCOUNTABILITY

One of the key benefits of joining a fitness class or group is the social support you gain.
1. ACCOUNTABILITY PARTNERS: When others expect you to show up, it's harder to skip workouts, keeping you consistent.
2. ENCOURAGEMENT AND CAMARADERIE: Sharing goals and progress with others fosters encouragement and a sense of belonging, making the weight loss journey less isolating.

48.4 OVERCOMING FITNESS ANXIETY

For beginners, joining a fitness class or group can feel intimidating. However, most classes are welcoming, and participants are often supportive of each other's progress.
1. START WITH BEGINNER-FRIENDLY Options: Look for classes labeled as beginner or introductory to ease Into the routine.
2. ATTEND WITH A FRIEND: Bringing someone you know can make the experience less daunting and more enjoyable.

48.5 STAYING CONSISTENT IN A FITNESS CLASS

Consistency is key to seeing results.
1. **CHOOSE A CLASS THAT FITS YOUR SCHEDULE:** Select a time and location that you can commit to regularly.
2. **SET CLEAR GOALS:** Whether it's improving endurance, strength, or flexibility, having goals helps maintain your focus.

48.6 THE LONG-TERM IMPACT OF GROUP FITNESS

Participating in a fitness class or group not only aids in weight loss but also fosters long-term health habits. You're more likely to stick to an active lifestyle when it's enjoyable and socially engaging.

By joining a fitness class or group, you tap into a network of support and expertise that makes achieving your health and fitness goals more attainable.

CHAPTER 49: USE HERBS AND SPICES FOR FLAVOR

49.1 THE POWER OF HERBS AND SPICES

Incorporating herbs and spices into your meals is a simple yet effective way to boost flavor without adding extra calories or unhealthy ingredients. Unlike salt, sugar, or fat, herbs and spices provide rich, complex flavors that can enhance any dish while also offering numerous health benefits. By experimenting with different combinations, you can transform your meals into flavorful, satisfying experiences that support your weight loss goals.

1. **FLAVOR WITHOUT THE CALORIES:** Herbs and spices add depth to your food without adding extra calories, sodium, or unhealthy fats.
2. **HEALTH BENEFITS:** Many herbs and spices are packed with antioxidants, anti-inflammatory properties, and metabolism-boosting compounds, which can aid in weight loss.

49.2 COMMON HERBS AND SPICES FOR WEIGHT LOSS

Certain herbs and spices are particularly beneficial for weight loss due to their ability to boost metabolism, reduce cravings, and support digestion. Here are some popular options to consider adding to your meals:

1. CAYENNE PEPPER: Known for its ability to increase metabolism and promote fat burning, cayenne pepper contains capsaicin, a compound that helps boost calorie burning.
2. GINGER: This spicy root helps improve digestion, reduce bloating, and can even reduce appetite. It's an excellent addition to both savory and sweet dishes.
3. CINNAMON: Known for its ability to stabilize blood sugar levels, cinnamon helps control cravings and prevents insulin spikes. It pairs well with smoothies, oatmeal, and baked goods.
4. TURMERIC: Containing the active compound curcumin, turmeric has powerful anti-inflammatory properties and supports fat metabolism. It's perfect for curries, soups, and even smoothies.
5. GARLIC: Garlic boosts the immune system and may help lower cholesterol levels. It also supports fat burning and aids digestion.

49.3 INCORPORATING HERBS AND SPICES INTO YOUR DIET

Adding herbs and spices to your meals doesn't require complex recipes or special cooking skills. Here are some simple ways to use them in your everyday meals:

1. SEASONING VEGETABLES: Instead of relying on butter or heavy sauces, season your vegetables with a variety of herbs like thyme, rosemary, or oregano. Roasting vegetables with olive oil and spices brings out their natural sweetness and flavor.
2. SPICE UP YOUR SALADS: Fresh herbs such as parsley, cilantro, and basil can elevate the flavor of salads. Try adding a handful of fresh herbs or a drizzle of lemon juice with a sprinkle of chili flakes.
3. FLAVORING PROTEINS: For grilled meats or fish, experiment with spices like cumin, paprika, or garlic powder. Marinate your protein with spices before cooking to infuse more flavor.
4. ADDING HERBS TO SMOOTHIES: Fresh herbs like mint or basil can be blended into smoothies for an added flavor boost. They add a refreshing taste without extra sugar or calories.
5. INFUSING WATER WITH HERBS AND SPICES: Try infusing your water with mint, cinnamon sticks, or ginger slices to add natural flavor without added sugars or artificial sweeteners.

49.4 BENEFITS BEYOND FLAVOR

In addition to enhancing the taste of your food, many herbs and spices provide a variety of health benefits that complement your weight loss efforts:

1. IMPROVED DIGESTION: Spices like ginger and peppermint can help improve digestion and reduce bloating, allowing you to feel lighter and more energized.
2. METABOLIC SUPPORT: Certain spices, such as cayenne pepper and turmeric, help improve metabolic function, making it easier to burn fat and maintain a healthy weight.
3. REDUCED INFLAMMATION: Chronic inflammation can hinder weight loss. Many herbs, including turmeric and garlic, have anti-inflammatory properties that can support a healthy body and mind.
4. APPETITE CONTROL: Some herbs and spices, like cinnamon and ginger, help curb appetite and stabilize blood sugar levels, preventing overeating and reducing cravings.

49.5 MAKING HERBS AND SPICES A HABIT

To truly benefit from the flavor and health advantages of herbs and spices, it's essential to make them a regular part of your meals.

1. KEEP THEM VISIBLE: Store your herbs and spices in an easily accessible place so you can easily grab them when preparing meals.
2. START SIMPLE: If you're new to using herbs and spices, start by adding a couple of your favorites to meals and gradually experiment with new combinations.
3. CREATE A SPICE BAR: Consider creating a spice rack or spice drawer in your kitchen with a variety of dried herbs, spices, and blends to encourage experimentation.
4. EXPLORE NEW RECIPES: Challenge yourself to try new recipes that incorporate herbs and spices you haven't used before. This will keep your meals exciting and flavorful.

49.6 CONCLUSION

Herbs and spices are a fantastic way to enhance your weight loss efforts while making your meals more flavorful and enjoyable. By incorporating a variety of herbs and spices into your cooking, you can reduce your reliance on unhealthy seasonings and make every meal a satisfying, flavorful experience. Whether you're boosting metabolism with cayenne pepper or improving digestion with ginger, herbs and spices offer a natural way to support your health and achieve your weight loss goals.

CHAPTER 50: LEVERAGE STRESS MANAGEMENT TO AVOID STRESS EATING

INTRODUCTION: Stress eating, also known as emotional eating, is a common challenge for many people trying to lose weight. When you're stressed, your body produces cortisol, a hormone that triggers cravings for comfort foods, especially those high in sugar, fat, and salt. Managing stress effectively can help you avoid this urge to overeat and support your weight loss goals. In this chapter, we'll explore techniques to manage stress and prevent stress eating.

50.1 UNDERSTANDING STRESS EATING: Stress eating is often an automatic response to difficult emotions or situations. When you're anxious, overwhelmed, or frustrated, food can provide a temporary sense of relief. Unfortunately, this can lead to overeating, particularly unhealthy foods, which contribute to weight gain. It's crucial to understand the connection between stress and eating patterns to manage it effectively.

50.2 THE ROLE OF CORTISOL IN STRESS EATING: Cortisol is a hormone produced by the adrenal glands in response to stress. When cortisol levels are high, your body signals the brain to seek out high-calorie foods to replenish energy quickly. This natural survival mechanism can cause you to crave junk food, but managing cortisol can prevent these cravings. By practicing stress-reduction techniques, you can lower cortisol levels and prevent stress-induced overeating.

50.3 PRACTICE MINDFULNESS AND MEDITATION: Mindfulness is the practice of staying present and aware of your thoughts and feelings without judgment. By practicing mindfulness, you can become more attuned to your emotions and physical hunger cues, rather than using food to cope with stress. Meditation helps calm the mind and reduces the overall stress response, making it less likely for you to turn to food for comfort. Dedicate a few minutes each day to mindfulness or meditation to reduce your stress levels and improve your relationship with food.

50.4 EXERCISE REGULARLY TO REDUCE STRESS: Physical activity is one of the most effective ways to manage stress and reduce the likelihood of stress eating. Exercise triggers the release of endorphins, which are natural mood elevators. Regular exercise helps manage cortisol levels and boosts overall well-being, making it less likely for you to use food as a coping mechanism. Aim for at least 30 minutes of moderate exercise most days of the week. Whether it's walking, yoga, or a more intense workout, find an activity you enjoy to keep stress at bay.

50.5 PRACTICE DEEP BREATHING EXERCISES: Deep breathing exercises can activate the parasympathetic nervous system, which helps the body relax and reduce stress. When you're feeling anxious or stressed, take a few minutes to breathe deeply. Inhale slowly through your nose for a count of four, hold for four, then exhale slowly through your mouth for a count of four. This simple technique can calm your mind and help you avoid reaching for food as a way to manage your emotions.

50.6 GET ENOUGH SLEEP: Lack of sleep can increase stress and lead to higher cortisol levels, which can trigger hunger and cravings for unhealthy foods. Prioritize sleep to support your weight loss goals and overall health. Aim for 7-9 hours of quality sleep each night. Create a calming bedtime routine, such as limiting screen time, dimming the lights, and practicing relaxation techniques to ensure a restful night's sleep.

50.7 IDENTIFY TRIGGERS AND FIND ALTERNATIVE COPING STRATEGIES:
Understanding what triggers your stress eating is crucial for managing the behavior. Is it work pressure, relationship challenges, or boredom? Once you identify your triggers, find healthier alternatives to deal with them. For example, if work stress leads to emotional eating, try taking a short walk, chatting with a friend, or practicing deep breathing instead. Developing these alternative coping strategies can help you stay on track with your weight loss journey.

50.8 USE SUPPORT SYSTEMS TO MANAGE STRESS: Having a strong support system is key to managing stress and avoiding stress eating. Talk to friends, family, or a therapist about your stressors. Sometimes, just verbalizing what's on your mind can alleviate the emotional burden. Additionally, joining a group or finding a workout buddy can provide encouragement and accountability, making it easier to stay on track with both stress management and weight loss.

CONCLUSION: Stress management plays a crucial role in preventing stress eating, which can hinder your weight loss efforts. By practicing mindfulness, engaging in regular physical activity, managing sleep, and using coping strategies, you can reduce the likelihood of turning to food when you're stressed. Incorporating these techniques into your daily routine will not only help you lose weight but also improve your overall health and emotional well-being. Focus on managing stress in a healthy way, and you'll feel more in control of both your emotions and your eating habits.

CHAPTER 51: AVOID HIGH-CALORIE BEVERAGES

51.1 INTRODUCTION
High-calorie beverages, such as sugary sodas, sweetened coffee drinks, and high-fat milkshakes, can quickly contribute to excess calorie intake. They often lack nutritional value and leave you feeling unsatisfied, prompting you to consume more food to compensate for the lack of fullness.

51.2 WHY YOU SHOULD AVOID HIGH-CALORIE BEVERAGES
These beverages are often packed with sugar and fats that add a significant number of calories without providing the necessary nutrients your body needs. The body processes liquid calories differently than solid food, meaning they don't provide the same feeling of

fullness, leading to overeating. High-calorie drinks can also cause blood sugar spikes, which can increase hunger and cravings.

51.3 HOW TO AVOID HIGH-CALORIE BEVERAGES

To reduce your calorie intake, switch to water, herbal teas, or black coffee with little or no sugar. If you crave flavor, try adding lemon or mint to your water. If you must drink juice, opt for freshly squeezed versions or low-calorie alternatives without added sugars.

CHAPTER 52: CHOOSE WHOLE GRAINS OVER REFINED GRAINS

52.1 INTRODUCTION

Whole grains are grains that retain all their original components, including the bran, germ, and endosperm. Examples include brown rice, whole wheat, quinoa, and oats. Refined grains, on the other hand, have been stripped of the bran and germ, such as white bread, white rice, and most breakfast cereals.

52.2 WHY WHOLE GRAINS ARE BETTER

Whole grains are rich in fiber, vitamins, and minerals, which are lost during the refining process. Fiber helps you feel full longer, reduces hunger cravings, and promotes healthy digestion. Whole grains have a lower glycemic index, which means they don't cause rapid spikes in blood sugar levels, making them a better option for weight loss and overall health.

52.3 HOW TO INCLUDE MORE WHOLE GRAINS IN YOUR DIET

Start by swapping white rice and pasta for brown rice, quinoa, or whole wheat pasta. Choose whole-grain bread instead of white bread and opt for oatmeal over sugary cereals. Gradually incorporate whole grains into your meals, making them a regular part of your diet.

CHAPTER 53: LIMIT PROCESSED MEATS

53.1 INTRODUCTION

Processed meats, such as sausages, hot dogs, bacon, and deli meats, are often high in unhealthy fats, sodium, and preservatives. These meats are linked to various health problems, including heart disease, diabetes, and high blood pressure.

53.2 WHY YOU SHOULD LIMIT PROCESSED MEATS

Processed meats are typically high in unhealthy fats and sodium, which can contribute to high cholesterol, heart disease, and other health issues. They are also often loaded with additives and preservatives, which can negatively impact your health in the long term. Studies have shown that consuming processed meats regularly is linked to an increased risk of weight gain and obesity.

53.3 HOW TO LIMIT PROCESSED MEATS

Instead of processed meats, choose lean cuts of fresh meats, such as chicken or turkey breast, or plant-based alternatives like beans, lentils, or tofu. Prepare your meals at home to have control over the ingredients, and limit the use of processed meats as much as possible.

CHAPTER 54: REPLACE SUGARY SNACKS WITH FRUIT

54.1 INTRODUCTION

Many snacks, such as cookies, candies, and chips, are high in sugar and empty calories. Replacing these sugary snacks with fruits can help curb your sweet tooth while providing essential nutrients.

54.2 WHY FRUITS ARE A HEALTHIER CHOICE

Fruits are naturally sweet and packed with vitamins, minerals, and fiber, which are beneficial for overall health. Unlike sugary snacks, fruits are lower in calories and provide lasting energy, keeping you full longer. The fiber content in fruits helps regulate digestion and maintains healthy blood sugar levels, preventing the spikes and crashes caused by sugary snacks.

54.3 HOW TO REPLACE SUGARY SNACKS WITH FRUIT

Keep a variety of fresh fruits available for quick, easy snacks. Berries, apples, oranges, and bananas are all excellent choices. If you're craving something sweeter, try dried fruit (without added sugar) or fruit smoothies made with yogurt or almond milk. Choose whole fruits over fruit juices for the added fiber benefits.

CHAPTER 55: AVOID HIGH-CALORIE SAUCES

55.1 INTRODUCTION
Many sauces, dressings, and condiments can add excessive calories to your meals without you even realizing it. These often contain unhealthy fats, sugars, and excess salt.

55.2 WHY YOU SHOULD AVOID HIGH-CALORIE SAUCES
High-calorie sauces can significantly increase the calorie content of an otherwise healthy meal. For example, creamy sauces, mayonnaise, and store-bought dressings can be packed with sugar, unhealthy fats, and preservatives. These can add up quickly and undermine your weight loss efforts.

55.3 HOW TO AVOID HIGH-CALORIE SAUCES
Opt for homemade, healthier versions of sauces and dressings using ingredients like olive oil, lemon juice, herbs, and vinegar. Use smaller amounts of sauce and focus on flavoring your meals with spices and herbs instead. When dining out, ask for dressings and sauces on the side to control how much you use.

CHAPTER 56: CHOOSE GRILLED OR BAKED FOODS

56.1 INTRODUCTION
Grilled and baked foods are healthier alternatives to fried foods, as they typically contain fewer calories and less fat. Grilling or baking preserves the flavor and texture of foods without the need for excessive oil or fat.

56.2 WHY GRILLED OR BAKED FOODS ARE BETTER
Frying adds unnecessary calories and unhealthy fats to foods, which can contribute to weight gain and other health issues. Grilling or baking, on the other hand, allows excess fats to drip away, resulting in a lower-calorie option. These methods also help retain more of the food's nutrients compared to frying.

56.3 HOW TO CHOOSE GRILLED OR BAKED FOODS

Whenever possible, choose grilled or baked items when dining out or preparing meals at home. For meats, opt for lean cuts like chicken breast or fish, and avoid deep-frying. You can also bake vegetables with a light drizzle of olive oil and seasoning to bring out their natural flavors.

CHAPTER 57: LIMIT YOUR INTAKE OF REFINED SUGAR

57.1 INTRODUCTION
Refined sugar, commonly found in candies, baked goods, sodas, and processed foods, is one of the main contributors to weight gain and health problems like diabetes and heart disease.

57.2 WHY YOU SHOULD LIMIT REFINED SUGAR
Refined sugar adds empty calories to your diet, leading to weight gain and poor health. It can cause blood sugar levels to spike, followed by a rapid crash, which increases cravings and leads to overeating. Regular consumption of refined sugar is linked to various chronic diseases, including obesity, type 2 diabetes, and metabolic syndrome.

57.3 HOW TO LIMIT REFINED SUGAR
Read food labels carefully to avoid hidden sugars in processed foods. Choose whole fruits for sweetness instead of sugary snacks or drinks. If you need to sweeten your meals or drinks, use natural sweeteners like honey or stevia, and always opt for moderation.

CHAPTER 58: EAT MORE SOUP

58.1 THE BENEFITS OF EATING SOUP

Soup is a highly nutritious, filling, and versatile meal option that supports weight loss in several ways. Firstly, it is hydrating and typically low in calories, making it an excellent choice for those seeking to manage their weight. The combination of liquid and fiber from vegetables can help fill you up, reducing the likelihood of overeating during meals.

Consuming soup can also aid in digestion and improve satiety due to the volume of liquid, helping you feel full longer.

58.2 HOW SOUP SUPPORTS WEIGHT LOSS

Eating a bowl of low-calorie, broth-based soup before a meal may help curb your appetite, leading to reduced calorie intake in the rest of the meal. By focusing on clear, vegetable-based soups, you can consume a nutrient-rich meal that is low in fat and high in fiber. The vegetables provide important vitamins and minerals without adding excessive calories. If you are using a base like broth or stock, you'll find that soup can be a satisfying and lower-calorie alternative to many other meal options.

58.3 TIPS FOR MAKING HEALTHY SOUPS

To make the most of soup for weight loss, avoid cream-based or overly rich soups, which can be calorie-dense. Focus on adding lean proteins like chicken or beans and bulk up your soup with fiber-rich vegetables like spinach, kale, and carrots. Adding legumes or whole grains can enhance the soup's nutritional value and keep you fuller for longer. Consider batch cooking your soups for meal prepping, as they can be stored for a few days in the refrigerator or frozen for later use. Always check the sodium content in store-bought soups and opt for low-sodium options when possible.

CHAPTER 59: CONTROL YOUR HUNGER WITH HEALTHY SNACKS

59.1 THE ROLE OF HEALTHY SNACKS IN WEIGHT MANAGEMENT
Snacking can either support or hinder your weight loss efforts, depending on your choices. When hunger strikes between meals, reaching for nutrient-dense, low-calorie snacks can prevent overeating during main meals. Healthy snacks help maintain energy levels and curb cravings, keeping your metabolism steady throughout the day.

59.2 IDEAL HEALTHY SNACKS
Opt for snacks like fresh fruits, vegetables with hummus, unsalted nuts, or Greek yogurt. These options are rich in fiber, protein, and healthy fats, which promote satiety and stabilize blood sugar levels. Avoid processed snacks high in sugar, salt, and unhealthy fats, as they can cause energy crashes and increased hunger.

59.3 SNACK PREPARATION TIPS

Prepare your snacks in advance to avoid impulsive, unhealthy choices. Portion out your snacks to avoid overeating, and always have them on hand at work or while traveling.

CHAPTER 60: EAT HIGH-VOLUME, LOW-CALORIE FOODS

60.1 UNDERSTANDING HIGH-VOLUME, LOW-CALORIE FOODS
High-volume, low-calorie foods are nutrient-dense but low in energy, meaning you can eat larger portions without consuming many calories. These include fruits, vegetables, and soups, which fill you up without exceeding your calorie budget.

60.2 BENEFITS OF HIGH-VOLUME FOODS
These foods help reduce hunger and promote satiety, making it easier to stick to your weight loss plan. By consuming high-volume foods, you can enjoy larger portions, which is psychologically satisfying while still losing weight.

60.3 HOW TO INCORPORATE THEM INTO MEALS
Start meals with a salad or vegetable soup to help control portions of higher-calorie foods. Bulk up dishes with vegetables and use fruits as a natural dessert.

CHAPTER 61: TRY YOGA OR PILATES FOR FLEXIBILITY

61.1 BENEFITS OF YOGA AND PILATES FOR WEIGHT LOSS
While these practices are not as calorie-intensive as cardio, they improve flexibility, balance, and mental focus, which indirectly support weight loss. Yoga and Pilates also help reduce stress, a common factor in overeating.

61.2 BUILDING STRENGTH AND ENDURANCE
Both exercises build core strength and improve posture. Stronger muscles increase resting metabolic rate, allowing your body to burn more calories even when at rest.

61.3 ADDING YOGA OR PILATES TO YOUR ROUTINE

Begin with beginner-friendly classes or online tutorials. Aim for consistency, incorporating 2–3 sessions per week. Over time, you'll notice increased flexibility and mental clarity.

CHAPTER 62: DRINK HERBAL TEAS

62.1 HERBAL TEAS FOR WEIGHT LOSS
Herbal teas like green tea, oolong, and peppermint offer numerous benefits for weight management. They are hydrating, low in calories, and contain compounds that may boost metabolism and aid fat oxidation.

62.2 APPETITE SUPPRESSION AND DETOXIFICATION
Some herbal teas, such as ginger or fennel, help suppress appetite and support digestion. Others like dandelion tea act as natural diuretics, reducing water retention and bloating.

62.3 HOW TO INCORPORATE HERBAL TEAS
Replace high-calorie beverages with herbal teas throughout the day. Enjoy them hot or cold, and avoid adding sugar or sweeteners to maximize their benefits.

CHAPTER 63: MAKE YOUR OWN SNACKS

63.1 THE IMPORTANCE OF HOMEMADE SNACKS
Homemade snacks give you control over ingredients, portion sizes, and calorie content. This eliminates the hidden sugars, salts, and unhealthy fats often found in store-bought snacks.

63.2 HEALTHY SNACK IDEAS
Prepare trail mix with nuts, seeds, and dried fruits, or bake kale chips for a crunchy, satisfying snack. Energy bars made with oats, honey, and nuts can serve as a convenient on-the-go option.

63.3 TIME-SAVING TIPS FOR SNACK PREP
Set aside time once a week to prepare and portion your snacks. Store them in airtight containers to keep them fresh and easily accessible.

CHAPTER 64: LIMIT TAKEOUT AND FAST FOOD

64.1 RISKS OF FREQUENT TAKEOUT
Takeout and fast food often contain high levels of unhealthy fats, sodium, and added sugars. Regular consumption can lead to weight gain and negatively impact overall health.

64.2 BENEFITS OF HOME-COOKED MEALS
Cooking at home allows you to choose healthier ingredients and control portion sizes. This ensures you consume balanced meals rich in nutrients, promoting sustainable weight loss.

64.3 STRATEGIES TO REDUCE TAKEOUT DEPENDENCY
Plan your meals and keep your pantry stocked with essentials. Batch cook and freeze meals for busy days. If you must order takeout, opt for healthier options like salads or grilled dishes.

CHAPTER 65: AVOID EXCESSIVE SALT

65.1 THE CONNECTION BETWEEN SALT AND WEIGHT GAIN
Excessive salt intake can lead to water retention, bloating, and an increase in blood pressure. While it doesn't directly cause fat gain, the added water weight can stall progress and make you feel heavier.

65.2 REDUCING SALT IN YOUR DIET
Flavor your meals with herbs, spices, and citrus instead of relying on salt. Be cautious with processed and prepackaged foods, as they often contain hidden sodium.

65.3 LONG-TERM BENEFITS OF LOW-SODIUM DIETS
A reduced-sodium diet not only supports weight loss but also lowers the risk of heart disease and hypertension. Over time, your taste buds will adapt, and you'll enjoy the natural flavors of foods.

CHAPTER 66: GET SUPPORT FROM FRIENDS AND FAMILY

66.1 THE IMPORTANCE OF SOCIAL SUPPORT

One of the key factors in achieving long-term weight loss success is having a strong support system. When you embark on a weight loss journey, the encouragement and understanding of friends and family can significantly increase your chances of success. Social support provides not only motivation and accountability but also emotional backing when faced with challenges. Studies show that those who have a supportive network tend to experience better outcomes in terms of weight loss and maintenance.

1. **ACCOUNTABILITY AND MOTIVATION:** Friends and family can help you stay on track by offering gentle reminders and celebrating your victories.
2. **EMOTIONAL ENCOURAGEMENT:** Weight loss can be an emotional rollercoaster, and having loved ones by your side provides comfort and reassurance during tough times.

66.2 HOW FRIENDS AND FAMILY CAN HELP

Involving your loved ones in your weight loss journey doesn't mean they have to be experts in fitness or nutrition. Their support can come in many different forms:

1. **JOINING YOU IN PHYSICAL ACTIVITY:** Having a walking or exercise buddy can make physical activity more enjoyable. Invite a friend or family member to go for walks, jog, or attend a fitness class together. Exercising with others helps you stay consistent and makes the experience more fun.
2. **ENCOURAGING HEALTHY EATING:** Sharing healthy meals or recipes with loved ones can make eating nutritious foods more enjoyable and less of a challenge. You can cook and enjoy healthy meals together, making it a bonding experience.
3. **PROVIDING MOTIVATIONAL SUPPORT:** When you're feeling discouraged, your friends and family can be a source of motivation. A few words of encouragement can reignite your determination and push you through moments of doubt.

4. CHEERING FOR YOUR SUCCESSES: Acknowledge your progress with your loved ones, no matter how small the achievement. Having people to celebrate your wins with makes the journey more rewarding and reinforces your commitment to your goals.

66.3 HOW TO ASK FOR SUPPORT

Sometimes, you may feel hesitant to ask for support, especially if you think others may not understand your goals. However, the more open and honest you are about your intentions, the more likely you'll receive the support you need. Here are some tips on how to ask for help from those closest to you:

1. COMMUNICATE YOUR GOALS: Be clear about what you're trying to achieve and why it's important to you. When your loved ones understand your goals, they'll be more likely to offer their support in ways that are meaningful to you.

2. BE SPECIFIC: Instead of a vague request like, "Please help me lose weight," try something more specific. For example, "It would mean a lot to me if you could join me for a 30-minute walk three times a week" or "Could you help me keep track of my meals by joining me in preparing healthy dinners?"

3. SET REALISTIC EXPECTATIONS: Let your loved ones know that you're not expecting perfection from yourself or them. Weight loss is a journey with ups and downs, and their support will help you get back on track after any setbacks.

4. EXPRESS GRATITUDE: Acknowledge and thank your friends and family for their support. Feeling appreciated can motivate them to continue helping you on your journey.

66.4 SUPPORT GROUPS AND ONLINE COMMUNITIES

In addition to your immediate circle, you can also find support through larger groups or online communities. These platforms allow you to connect with people who are on similar journeys and share experiences, challenges, and success stories.

1. JOINING A SUPPORT GROUP: Many communities offer in-person or online weight loss support groups where you can exchange tips, offer encouragement, and receive advice from others. Support groups provide a sense of camaraderie, and knowing you're not alone in your struggles can be reassuring.

2. ONLINE COMMUNITIES: Online forums and social media groups can also provide valuable support. Joining a Facebook group, subscribing to weight loss blogs, or participating in online challenges can keep you engaged and motivated.

66.5 HANDLING NEGATIVE REACTIONS

While most friends and family will be supportive, not everyone will understand or encourage your journey. It's important to handle negative reactions with confidence and kindness.

1. SET BOUNDARIES: If someone offers unsolicited advice or expresses doubt about your goals, politely set boundaries by explaining your commitment to your health and well-being.

2. STAY FOCUSED: Remember that weight loss is a personal journey. Negative comments or lack of support can be discouraging, but it's important to stay focused on your reasons for embarking on this journey.

3. SURROUND YOURSELF WITH POSITIVITY: If you encounter negativity from certain people, focus on those who support you and uplift your spirits. Seek out relationships that nurture and encourage your success.

66.6 BENEFITS OF HAVING A SUPPORT SYSTEM

Having a strong network of support can make all the difference in your weight loss journey. The benefits are numerous:

1. ENHANCED MOTIVATION: Regular encouragement from your support system will keep you motivated, even when the progress seems slow.

2. REDUCED STRESS: Knowing you have people to lean on reduces the stress that can come with dieting or exercising alone.

3. INCREASED CHANCES OF SUCCESS: Studies show that those who have a supportive network are more likely to lose weight and maintain their progress long-term.

66.7 CONCLUSION

Achieving weight loss goals is easier when you have the support of friends and family. Their encouragement, help with physical activity, and emotional backing can make the process more enjoyable and effective. By being open about your goals, asking for specific help, and joining supportive groups, you can create a strong network that boosts your chances of success. Remember, you don't have to do it alone—share your journey, and let others help you stay on track.

CHAPTER 67: USE FERMENTED FOODS TO BOOST IMMUNE FUNCTION

A strong immune system is essential for maintaining overall health and wellness, and one powerful way to support your immunity is by including fermented foods in your diet. Fermented foods are rich in probiotics, which are beneficial bacteria that help maintain a healthy gut microbiome. A balanced gut is crucial for immune function, as a significant portion of your immune system resides in the gut. In this chapter, we'll explore how fermented foods can enhance your immune health and how to incorporate them into your diet.

67.1 UNDERSTANDING FERMENTED FOODS AND THEIR BENEFITS

Fermentation is a natural process in which microorganisms such as bacteria, yeasts, and molds break down food sugars and starches. This process not only preserves foods but also enhances their nutritional profile. Fermented foods are particularly beneficial for gut health, and in turn, they can help support a strong immune system. Some key benefits of fermented foods include:

*IMPROVED DIGESTION: Fermented foods contain live probiotics, which help balance the gut microbiome and improve digestion. A healthy gut can prevent digestive issues like bloating, constipation, and indigestion.

*ENHANCED NUTRIENT ABSORPTION: Probiotics improve the absorption of essential nutrients, such as vitamins and minerals, by aiding in the breakdown of food.

*IMMUNE SYSTEM SUPPORT: About 70% of your immune system is housed in the gut. Probiotics found in fermented foods help regulate immune responses and enhance the body's ability to fight off infections.

*REDUCED INFLAMMATION: The beneficial bacteria in fermented foods can reduce inflammation in the body, which is linked to a variety of chronic conditions, including autoimmune diseases and allergies.

67.2 TYPES OF FERMENTED FOODS FOR IMMUNE SUPPORT

There are many fermented foods to choose from, each offering different types of probiotics and other beneficial nutrients. Below are some of the best fermented foods to incorporate into your diet to boost immune function:

67.2.1 YOGURT

Yogurt is one of the most well-known fermented foods, and it's rich in probiotics like Lactobacillus and Bifidobacterium. These probiotics can help balance the gut microbiome, which plays a direct role in regulating immune function. Look for plain, unsweetened yogurt to avoid excess sugar that can undermine its health benefits.

67.2.2 KEFIR

Kefir is a fermented dairy beverage similar to yogurt but with a wider variety of probiotics. It contains beneficial yeast and bacteria that promote a healthy gut. Kefir is also a good source of protein, calcium, and vitamin D, all of which contribute to immune health.

67.2.3 KIMCHI

Kimchi, a traditional Korean side dish made from fermented vegetables (primarily cabbage), is rich in probiotics, vitamins A, B, and C, and antioxidants. It also contains Lactobacillus bacteria, which helps with digestion and supports the immune system. The fermentation process also enhances its anti-inflammatory properties.

67.2.4 SAUERKRAUT

Sauerkraut is another fermented vegetable, typically made from cabbage. It's rich in probiotics, fiber, and vitamin C. The fermentation process also enhances the bioavailability of nutrients, making it easier for the body to absorb essential minerals like iron and magnesium. Regular consumption of sauerkraut can support gut health, which in turn helps regulate immune responses.

67.2.5 MISO

Miso is a fermented paste made from soybeans, salt, and koji mold. It's a staple in Japanese cuisine and is often used in soups and sauces. Miso contains probiotics that support gut health, and it's also rich in antioxidants, vitamins, and minerals. Including miso in your diet can boost your immune system and promote digestive health.

67.2.6 TEMPEH

Tempeh is a fermented soybean product that is rich in protein, fiber, and probiotics. It also contains various vitamins and minerals, such as iron and magnesium. The fermentation process makes the soy protein in tempeh easier to digest, promoting gut health and immune function.

67.2.7 KOMBUCHA

Kombucha is a fermented tea that contains beneficial bacteria, yeast, and polyphenols. It has antioxidant properties that can support immune health. Kombucha also contains B vitamins and organic acids that help detoxify the body, reduce inflammation, and support a healthy gut microbiome.

67.3 HOW FERMENTED FOODS SUPPORT IMMUNE FUNCTION

The relationship between the gut microbiome and the immune system is complex but vital. The gut contains trillions of microbes that communicate with the immune system, and these microbes play a significant role in immune responses. Fermented foods help maintain a healthy balance of good bacteria in the gut, which can:

*ENHANCE IMMUNE RESPONSE: Probiotics in fermented foods can increase the production of antibodies and immune cells, which help the body fight infections more effectively.

*REGULATE INFLAMMATION: A balanced gut microbiome can reduce chronic inflammation, which is linked to numerous health problems, including autoimmune diseases and allergies.

*PREVENT PATHOGEN OVERGROWTH: Fermented foods help prevent the overgrowth of harmful bacteria and pathogens in the gut, which can weaken the immune system.

*PROMOTE HEALTHY GUT LINING: Fermented foods promote the production of beneficial compounds that help maintain the integrity of the gut lining, preventing "leaky gut," a condition linked to autoimmune disorders.

67.4 HOW TO INCORPORATE FERMENTED FOODS INTO YOUR DIET

Incorporating fermented foods into your daily diet is easier than you might think. Here are some practical tips:

*ADD YOGURT TO BREAKFAST: Enjoy a bowl of yogurt with fruits, nuts, or seeds as a healthy breakfast option.

*USE SAUERKRAUT AND KIMCHI AS TOPPINGS: Add sauerkraut or kimchi to sandwiches, wraps, or salads for a tangy, probiotic-rich boost.

*DRINK KEFIR OR KOMBUCHA: Swap sugary beverages with kefir or kombucha to hydrate and support your gut health.

*INCLUDE MISO IN SOUPS AND SAUCES: Add miso to soups, stews, and stir-fries for a flavorful, immune-boosting addition.

*USE TEMPEH AS A MEAT SUBSTITUTE: Tempeh can be used as a plant-based protein in stir-fries, sandwiches, and salads.

67.5 CONCLUSION

Fermented foods are an excellent addition to your diet if you want to boost your immune function and support overall health. By including probiotic-rich foods like yogurt, kefir, kimchi, and sauerkraut in your daily meals, you can enhance your gut health, reduce inflammation, and strengthen your immune system. Whether you're looking to prevent illness or simply improve your digestive health, fermented foods are a delicious and nutritious way to promote a healthy, well-balanced body.

CHAPTER 68: OPT FOR DARK CHOCOLATE INSTEAD OF MILK CHOCOLATE

68.1 THE BENEFITS OF DARK CHOCOLATE

Dark chocolate, especially varieties with 70% cocoa or more, has been shown to have various health benefits. It's rich in antioxidants and can help reduce cravings for sweet, processed snacks. Dark chocolate also has less sugar than milk chocolate, making it a healthier option for weight loss.

68.2 HOW TO ENJOY DARK CHOCOLATE IN MODERATION

While dark chocolate has benefits, it should still be eaten in moderation. A small square (around 1 ounce) is sufficient to satisfy your sweet tooth without overindulging. You can also combine it with healthy snacks like nuts or fruits to enhance its benefits and curb cravings.

68.3 AVOID CHOCOLATE PRODUCTS WITH FILLERS

Many chocolate products on the market contain additives, sugar, and artificial flavoring. Opt for high-quality, pure dark chocolate that contains minimal ingredients for the best nutritional benefits.

CHAPTER 69: MAKE HEALTHY SWAPS FOR COMFORT FOODS

69.1 WHY SWAPPING IS ESSENTIAL FOR WEIGHT LOSS

Comfort foods, like pizza, fried foods, and creamy pastas, are often loaded with calories and unhealthy fats. However, by making healthy swaps, you can enjoy the flavors you love while staying on track with your weight loss goals. Swapping ingredients allows you to satisfy cravings without compromising on nutrition.

69.2 HEALTHY SWAPS YOU CAN MAKE

*PIZZA: Try a cauliflower crust or use whole wheat dough, topped with lean proteins and plenty of veggies.

*FRIED FOODS: Swap deep frying for baking or air frying to reduce calories and fat content.

*PASTA: Choose spiralized vegetables like zucchini or butternut squash instead of regular pasta. Alternatively, opt for whole grain pasta.

*CREAMY SAUCES: Replace heavy cream with Greek yogurt or avocado for a creamy texture without the calories.

69.3 THE IMPORTANCE OF CREATIVITY IN SWAPS

The key to successfully swapping comfort foods is creativity. Experiment with healthier alternatives until you find what works best for your taste preferences.

CHAPTER 70: ADD MORE FIBER TO YOUR DIET

70.1 WHY FIBER IS CRUCIAL FOR WEIGHT LOSS

Fiber is an essential nutrient that helps keep you feeling full and satisfied, which can help reduce overeating. It also aids digestion and supports gut health. Fiber-rich foods such as vegetables, fruits, legumes, and whole grains promote regular bowel movements and reduce bloating, contributing to a more comfortable and effective weight loss journey.

70.2 HOW TO INCREASE FIBER IN YOUR DIET

To increase your fiber intake, focus on incorporating more plant-based foods into your meals. Eat whole grains like quinoa, brown rice, and oats instead of refined grains. Include more vegetables, fruits, beans, and legumes in your dishes. You can also snack on fiber-rich foods like almonds, apples, and carrots.

70.3 TIPS FOR SUCCESS

Make fiber a priority at every meal. For example, start your day with a fiber-packed breakfast such as oatmeal with chia seeds or fruit. When preparing meals, aim to fill half your plate with vegetables to increase fiber content and reduce the temptation to overeat.

CHAPTER 71: KEEP YOUR STRESS UNDER CONTROL

71.1 THE LINK BETWEEN STRESS AND WEIGHT GAIN

Chronic stress can negatively affect your weight loss goals. It triggers the release of cortisol, a hormone that promotes fat storage, especially around the abdomen. Stress can also lead to emotional eating, where you turn to comfort foods to cope with overwhelming feelings.

71.2 STRESS-REDUCING TECHNIQUES

To keep stress under control, try incorporating relaxation practices into your daily routine. Techniques like deep breathing, meditation, yoga, and mindfulness can help lower stress levels and prevent overeating. Regular exercise is another great way to manage stress while improving your mood and boosting your metabolism.

71.3 SEEK SUPPORT WHEN NEEDED

If stress becomes overwhelming, consider seeking professional support from a therapist or counselor. Managing stress effectively can have a profound impact on your weight loss progress and overall health.

CHAPTER 72: INCORPORATE STRENGTH TRAINING TO BUILD MUSCLE

72.1 THE BENEFITS OF STRENGTH TRAINING

Strength training is a crucial component of any weight loss program. Building muscle increases your resting metabolic rate, meaning you burn more calories even when you're not exercising. It also helps to tone and sculpt your body, giving you a leaner appearance.

72.2 STRENGTH TRAINING EXERCISES TO TRY

Incorporate exercises like squats, lunges, push-ups, and deadlifts into your routine. Resistance exercises using free weights, resistance bands, or bodyweight exercises can be highly effective. Aim for at least two to three strength training sessions per week, with a focus on major muscle groups.

72.3 COMBINE STRENGTH TRAINING WITH CARDIO

For optimal results, combine strength training with cardiovascular exercises. This combination will help you burn fat while building lean muscle, ultimately supporting your weight loss goals.

CHAPTER 73: SKIP SUGARY CEREALS FOR BREAKFAST

73.1 WHY SUGARY CEREALS ARE A POOR CHOICE

Many popular breakfast cereals are loaded with refined sugars, which can cause blood sugar spikes followed by crashes. This can leave you feeling hungry soon after eating and may lead to overeating later in the day. Additionally, sugary cereals offer little nutritional value and can set you back in your weight loss efforts.

73.2 HEALTHY ALTERNATIVES FOR BREAKFAST

Opt for whole grain cereals or oats that are low in sugar. You can add your own natural sweetness with fresh fruits like berries, bananas, or apples. For a protein boost, consider adding a handful of nuts, seeds, or Greek yogurt.

73.3 PREPARE YOUR BREAKFAST THE NIGHT BEFORE

To make healthy breakfasts more convenient, prepare your meals the night before. Overnight oats or smoothie packs are great options that can be quickly grabbed in the morning.

CHAPTER 74: EAT MORE LOW-FAT DAIRY PRODUCTS

74.1 THE ADVANTAGES OF LOW-FAT DAIRY

Low-fat dairy products such as yogurt, milk, and cheese provide important nutrients like calcium, protein, and vitamins without the added fat and calories found in full-fat versions. They are also easier to digest for many people, and their protein content helps you feel fuller for longer.

74.2 TIPS FOR INCORPORATING LOW-FAT DAIRY

Replace full-fat dairy with low-fat alternatives whenever possible. Choose skim or 1% milk, fat-free yogurt, and reduced-fat cheese. You can also enjoy plant-based options like almond milk or coconut yogurt, which are low in fat and often fortified with calcium and vitamins.

74.3 BALANCE DAIRY WITH OTHER NUTRIENTS

While dairy is an important part of a balanced diet, don't forget to include other nutrient-rich foods like vegetables, lean proteins, and whole grains to maintain a well-rounded diet.

CHAPTER 75: INCLUDE HEALTHY SNACKS BETWEEN MEALS

75.1 THE ROLE OF HEALTHY SNACKS

Healthy snacks are an important tool for managing hunger and stabilizing blood sugar levels between meals. When you are hungry, your body craves quick energy, and choosing a healthy snack ensures that you stay on track with your weight loss goals. By opting for nutrient-dense snacks, you reduce the temptation to binge on unhealthy foods later in the day.

75.2 IDEAL SNACK CHOICES

Choose snacks that combine protein, fiber, and healthy fats. Some examples include:

*A handful of mixed nuts and seeds.

*Sliced veggies with hummus or guacamole.

*Greek yogurt with fresh berries.

*A small portion of cottage cheese with pineapple.

*Hard-boiled eggs. These snacks are not only satisfying but also provide essential nutrients that support weight loss and overall health.

75.3 SCHEDULE YOUR SNACKS

Plan your snacks just as you would your meals. Avoid mindlessly snacking throughout the day, as it can lead to overeating. Instead, have a set time for snacks to prevent you from reaching for junk food when hunger strikes unexpectedly.

CHAPTER 76: REPLACE SODA WITH SPARKLING WATER

76.1 THE IMPACT OF SODA ON YOUR HEALTH

Soda is a staple in many diets, but it comes with significant health risks. Loaded with sugar, artificial flavors, and empty calories, regular soda consumption can lead to weight gain, increased blood sugar levels, and a higher risk of chronic conditions like type 2 diabetes, heart disease, and obesity. Even diet sodas, though calorie-free, often contain artificial sweeteners that may disrupt your metabolism and trigger cravings for sweet foods.

1. HIGH SUGAR CONTENT: A single can of regular soda contains about 39 grams of sugar, far exceeding the recommended daily intake for most adults.
2. EMPTY CALORIES: Soda provides no essential nutrients, meaning the calories consumed are not beneficial to your body.
3. HEALTH RISKS: Regular soda consumption is linked to various health problems, including weight gain and increased risk of chronic diseases.

76.2 WHY SWITCH TO SPARKLING WATER

Replacing soda with sparkling water is a simple yet effective step toward better health. Sparkling water offers the same fizzy satisfaction without the harmful additives found in soda. It's a refreshing, hydrating, and low-calorie alternative that can help you curb your soda cravings while supporting your weight loss goals.

1. ZERO SUGAR AND CALORIES: Unlike soda, sparkling water contains no sugar or calories, making it a guilt-free option.
2. HYDRATION BENEFITS: Sparkling water hydrates as effectively as still water, keeping your body well-functioning.
3. VARIETY OF FLAVORS: Many brands offer naturally flavored sparkling waters without added sugars or artificial sweeteners, giving you the option to enjoy a range of tastes.

76.3 HOW TO MAKE THE SWITCH

Transitioning from soda to sparkling water doesn't have to be difficult. With the right approach, you can reduce your soda consumption and enjoy the benefits of a healthier beverage choice.

1. START GRADUALLY: If you're a regular soda drinker, begin by replacing one soda a day with sparkling water. Gradually increase the number of times you opt for sparkling water until soda is no longer part of your routine.
2. EXPERIMENT WITH FLAVORS: To keep things interesting, try different flavors of sparkling water. Look for options infused with natural fruit essences, such as lemon, lime, berry, or cucumber. You can also add a splash of freshly squeezed juice for a touch of sweetness without the added sugar.
3. MAKE IT A HABIT: Incorporate sparkling water into your daily routine. For example, have a glass with your meals or keep a bottle at your desk to sip throughout the day.

76.4 BENEFITS OF SWITCHING TO SPARKLING WATER

Making the switch from soda to sparkling water offers numerous health and lifestyle benefits:

1. WEIGHT MANAGEMENT: Cutting out sugary sodas reduces your calorie intake, helping you maintain a healthy weight or shed excess pounds.
2. BETTER DENTAL HEALTH: Sparkling water is far less acidic than soda, reducing the risk of tooth decay and enamel erosion.
3. IMPROVED BLOOD SUGAR LEVELS: Eliminating sugary drinks helps stabilize your blood sugar, lowering the risk of developing type 2 diabetes.
4. REDUCED RISK OF CHRONIC DISEASES: By avoiding the excessive sugar and artificial ingredients in soda, you lower your chances of developing heart disease, metabolic syndrome, and other health issues.

76.5 DEALING WITH CRAVINGS

It's natural to experience cravings for soda, especially if it's been a part of your daily routine for years. Here's how to handle those cravings effectively:

1. KEEP SPARKLING WATER HANDY: Always have sparkling water within reach to satisfy your craving for something fizzy.
2. INFUSE WITH FRUITS OR HERBS: Enhance the flavor of your sparkling water with slices of citrus, berries, or fresh mint leaves. This makes it more appealing and satisfying.
3. REMIND YOURSELF OF THE BENEFITS: When cravings strike, think about the health benefits you're gaining by choosing sparkling water over soda.

76.6 SPARKLING WATER IN SOCIAL SETTINGS

Social situations often involve soda, whether it's at parties, restaurants, or gatherings. Here's how to stay committed to your sparkling water habit without feeling left out:

1. BRING YOUR OWN: If you're attending a gathering, bring a few bottles of your favorite sparkling water to share.
2. REQUEST SPARKLING WATER: At restaurants, ask for sparkling water instead of soda. Many establishments offer it as an alternative.
3. GET CREATIVE WITH MOCKTAILS: Use sparkling water as a base for mocktails. Combine it with fruit juices, herbs, and ice to create a refreshing and festive drink.

76.7 CONCLUSION

Replacing soda with sparkling water is a simple yet powerful change that can have a significant impact on your health. By eliminating the excessive sugar, calories, and artificial ingredients found in soda, you can enjoy a fizzy and refreshing beverage that supports your weight loss and overall well-being. Start gradually, experiment with flavors, and embrace this healthier alternative as part of your daily routine.

CHAPTER 77: DRINK WATER BEFORE MEALS

77.1 WHY WATER IS ESSENTIAL FOR WEIGHT LOSS

Drinking water before meals helps control hunger and prevents overeating. Studies have shown that consuming water before meals can help reduce the amount of food you eat, leading to fewer calories consumed. It also aids in digestion and ensures that your body is well-hydrated, which is essential for overall health.

77.2 HOW MUCH WATER SHOULD YOU DRINK?

Aim to drink at least 16-20 ounces (about 500-600 ml) of water about 30 minutes before a meal. This not only helps curb appetite but also ensures that your body is properly hydrated before you begin eating.

77.3 ADD FLAVOR IF NECESSARY

If plain water feels too bland, you can add a slice of lemon, cucumber, or mint for a refreshing twist. Herbal teas are also a good alternative for added flavor and hydration without added calories.

CHAPTER 78: INCLUDE LEAN PROTEINS IN EVERY MEAL

78.1 THE IMPORTANCE OF PROTEIN IN WEIGHT LOSS

Protein plays a vital role in weight loss as it increases feelings of fullness and boosts metabolism. It also helps preserve muscle mass while you lose fat, which is crucial for long-term weight management. Lean protein sources are lower in fat and calories, making them an excellent choice for anyone looking to lose weight.

78.2 SOURCES OF LEAN PROTEIN

Some healthy sources of lean protein include:

*Skinless poultry (chicken or turkey)

*Fish (salmon, tuna, cod)

*Legumes (lentils, beans, chickpeas)

*Tofu and tempeh

*Low-fat dairy (Greek yogurt, cottage cheese)

*Lean cuts of red meat (sirloin, flank steak)

78.3 HOW TO INTEGRATE PROTEIN INTO YOUR DIET

Make sure to include a source of protein in every meal. For example, add chicken to salads, eggs to breakfast, or beans to soups. Including protein-rich snacks, such as hard-boiled eggs or a protein bar, is also a great way to curb hunger.

CHAPTER 79: PLAN YOUR MEALS IN ADVANCE

79.1 THE BENEFITS OF MEAL PLANNING

Meal planning is essential for weight loss as it helps prevent impulse eating and ensures that you are consuming balanced, healthy meals throughout the week. By planning your meals ahead of time, you can create a grocery list, reduce food waste, and stick to portion control. It also helps you make smarter food choices and saves time during the week.

79.2 HOW TO PLAN YOUR MEALS

Start by creating a weekly meal plan that includes breakfast, lunch, dinner, and snacks. Focus on including a variety of nutrient-dense foods, such as vegetables, fruits, whole grains, lean proteins, and healthy fats. Pre-cook or prepare ingredients in bulk, so you can easily assemble your meals on busy days.

79.3 STAY FLEXIBLE

While it's important to stick to your meal plan, allow for some flexibility. Life is unpredictable, and you may need to adjust meals based on unexpected events. The key is to plan ahead but also remain adaptable.

CHAPTER 80: EAT SLOWLY AND MINDFULLY

80.1 WHY MINDFUL EATING IS IMPORTANT

Mindful eating involves paying attention to the experience of eating – the taste, texture, and smell of food. By eating slowly and being aware of your body's hunger and fullness signals, you can prevent overeating. It also allows you to fully enjoy your food, reducing the likelihood of cravings later.

80.2 HOW TO PRACTICE MINDFUL EATING

To practice mindful eating, take the time to sit down for each meal without distractions. Focus on each bite, chew thoroughly, and savor the flavors. Put your fork down between bites and listen to your body. If you feel full, stop eating. This can help prevent overeating and promote healthier portion sizes.

80.3 AVOID EATING IN FRONT OF SCREENS

Eating while distracted, such as watching TV or scrolling through your phone, can lead to overeating. Make your meals a time to relax and be present, so you can tune in to your body's signals and enjoy your food more.

CHAPTER 81: STAY CONSISTENT WITH EXERCISE

81.1 WHY CONSISTENCY MATTERS

Consistency is key when it comes to weight loss. Engaging in regular physical activity, including both cardio and strength training exercises, helps burn calories and build muscle, which in turn supports fat loss. Skipping workouts or only exercising sporadically can hinder progress.

81.2 EXERCISE ROUTINES TO TRY

Aim to include a mix of activities in your weekly routine:

*CARDIO: Walking, running, cycling, swimming, or dancing.

*STRENGTH TRAINING: Resistance exercises using weights, resistance bands, or bodyweight exercises like push-ups and squats.

*FLEXIBILITY AND BALANCE: Yoga, Pilates, or stretching exercises to improve flexibility and reduce the risk of injury.

81.3 STICKING TO A SCHEDULE

Set a regular exercise schedule and stick to it. Whether you prefer working out in the morning or evening, make exercise a priority by scheduling it in your calendar. Consistency is the key to seeing lasting results.

CHAPTER 82: DRINK GREEN SMOOTHIES FOR DETOX AND ENERGY

INTRODUCTION:
Green smoothies have gained popularity in recent years as a powerhouse drink packed with essential nutrients that promote detoxification and boost energy levels. If you're looking to enhance your weight loss journey, incorporating green smoothies into your diet can offer a refreshing, nutritious, and effective way to support your overall health. These nutrient-dense drinks are made by blending leafy greens, fruits, and various superfoods, giving you a delicious yet powerful way to nourish your body.

1. THE BENEFITS OF GREEN SMOOTHIES

Green smoothies are not only an excellent way to support your weight loss goals but they also have multiple health benefits. Here are a few reasons why you should include green smoothies in your routine:

*DETOXIFICATION: The high fiber content from leafy greens such as spinach, kale, or arugula helps to cleanse your digestive system, flush out toxins, and promote regular bowel movements. This process helps rid your body of harmful substances and supports optimal health.

*BOOSTS ENERGY LEVELS: Green smoothies provide a natural energy boost. With ingredients like spinach, kale, and chia seeds, which are rich in vitamins, minerals, and antioxidants, they help combat fatigue and increase stamina.

*SUPPORTS WEIGHT LOSS: Green smoothies are low in calories but high in essential nutrients, which makes them a great option for filling you up without overloading you with empty calories. The fiber helps to keep you feeling full longer and prevents overeating.

*IMPROVES DIGESTION: The ingredients in green smoothies, such as ginger or aloe vera, aid digestion by soothing the stomach and promoting gut health. A healthy gut is essential for nutrient absorption, which ultimately supports your overall well-being.

2. KEY INGREDIENTS FOR A GREEN SMOOTHIE

To maximize the benefits of your green smoothie, choose ingredients that provide a balanced mixture of vitamins, minerals, and fiber. Here are some key components to consider:

*LEAFY GREENS: Spinach, kale, collard greens, and arugula are excellent sources of vitamins A, C, and K, as well as iron and magnesium. These greens are low in calories but packed with fiber and antioxidants.

*FRUITS: Adding fruits like apples, bananas, mangoes, and berries helps to sweeten the smoothie while providing additional vitamins, antioxidants, and fiber. Fruits also make the smoothie more palatable for those who may be new to green smoothies.

*HEALTHY FATS: Avocados, chia seeds, flaxseeds, or almond butter can add healthy fats, which help keep you feeling full longer and assist in nutrient absorption. Healthy fats also support brain function and overall cardiovascular health.

*SUPERFOODS: Consider adding superfoods like spirulina, chlorella, wheatgrass, or matcha powder to your smoothie for an extra boost of nutrients. These ingredients can help detoxify your body, improve digestion, and provide energy.

*LIQUID BASE: Use water, coconut water, almond milk, or any other low-calorie liquid to blend your smoothie. For a creamier texture, unsweetened coconut milk or oat milk can be a great choice.

*BOOSTERS: Adding ingredients like ginger, turmeric, lemon juice, or apple cider vinegar can enhance detoxification and digestion. These ingredients are known for their anti-inflammatory and immune-boosting properties.

3. HOW TO MAKE THE PERFECT GREEN SMOOTHIE

Making a green smoothie is simple and can be customized based on your preferences. Follow these steps to create your own delicious and nutritious drink:

1. PICK YOUR GREENS: Start by selecting your leafy greens. For beginners, spinach or baby kale is a great choice because they have a mild flavor. For a more robust taste, try arugula or Swiss chard.

2. ADD FRUITS: Add your favorite fruits to the blender. Aim for about 1-2 cups of fruit, depending on how sweet you want your smoothie to be. A banana is great for creaminess, while berries are loaded with antioxidants.

3. INCORPORATE HEALTHY FATS: Add 1 tablespoon of chia seeds, flaxseeds, or half an avocado to provide a healthy fat source. This will help keep you satisfied and promote proper nutrient absorption.

4. ADD A LIQUID BASE: Pour in 1-2 cups of your chosen liquid. Start with a small amount, as you can always add more for a thinner consistency.

5. INCLUDE SUPERFOODS AND BOOSTERS: Sprinkle in a teaspoon of your favorite superfoods or boosters like spirulina, ginger, turmeric, or cinnamon. These will enhance the nutritional value of your smoothie.

6. BLEND AND ENJOY: Blend everything together until smooth. If the consistency is too thick, add a bit more liquid until you reach your desired texture.

4. TIPS FOR SUCCESS

*START SLOW: If you're new to green smoothies, start with a small portion and gradually increase the quantity as your body adjusts to the change in diet.

*MIX UP YOUR GREENS: While spinach is a popular choice, rotating different greens can prevent taste fatigue and provide a broader range of nutrients.

*PRE-PACK YOUR SMOOTHIE: For a quick and convenient option, pre-pack your greens and fruits in freezer bags so you can simply toss them into the blender in the morning.

*AVOID OVERLOADING ON SUGAR: While fruits add sweetness, try to limit high-sugar fruits (like pineapples) to maintain a balanced smoothie that's not too high in calories.

*USE ORGANIC INGREDIENTS: Whenever possible, opt for organic greens, fruits, and superfoods to avoid pesticides and chemicals.

5. CONCLUSION

Green smoothies are an excellent addition to any weight loss plan. By incorporating nutrient-dense, detoxifying ingredients into your daily routine, you can increase your energy levels, enhance digestion, and support your body's natural detoxification process. The best part is that green smoothies are highly customizable, meaning you can experiment with different flavors and ingredients to keep things fresh and exciting. So, why not give green smoothies a try and reap the countless benefits they offer for your health and well-being?

CHAPTER 83: INCORPORATE MORE FRUITS AND VEGETABLES

83.1 THE BENEFITS OF FRUITS AND VEGETABLES

Fruits and vegetables are low in calories but packed with essential vitamins, minerals, and fiber. They promote satiety, helping you feel full while consuming fewer calories. Including more fruits and vegetables in your diet is an excellent strategy for losing weight and improving overall health.

83.2 HOW TO EAT MORE FRUITS AND VEGETABLES

Aim to fill half of your plate with vegetables and fruits at each meal. Add them to smoothies, salads, soups, and snacks. Keep a variety of fruits and vegetables on hand, so you have easy access to healthy options throughout the day.

83.3 FOCUS ON COLORFUL VARIETY

Eating a variety of colors ensures that you get a wide range of nutrients. Try to include different colored vegetables and fruits, such as leafy greens, peppers, berries, oranges, and purple eggplant, to maximize your nutrient intake.

CHAPTER 84: CHOOSE THE RIGHT SUPPLEMENTS TO SUPPORT WEIGHT LOSS

84.1 INTRODUCTION TO WEIGHT LOSS SUPPLEMENTS

When embarking on a weight loss journey, it's important to remember that supplements are not magic solutions. Instead, they serve as tools to enhance the effects of a balanced diet and regular exercise. Choosing the right supplements can provide nutritional support, boost metabolism, and help you stay on track with your weight loss goals. This chapter will explore some of the most effective and scientifically-backed weight loss supplements, how they work, and how to incorporate them into your routine safely.

84.2 COMMON TYPES OF WEIGHT LOSS SUPPLEMENTS

There are several types of supplements that can aid weight loss. Understanding the role of each can help you decide which might be best for your specific needs:

1. FAT BURNERS: These supplements typically contain a combination of ingredients that help to increase your body's ability to burn fat. Popular fat-burning ingredients include caffeine, green tea extract, and CLA (Conjugated Linoleic Acid). These compounds work by increasing thermogenesis, the process by which your body generates heat, burning calories in the process.

2. APPETITE SUPPRESSANTS: Appetite suppressants help reduce the sensation of hunger, making it easier to stick to a calorie-controlled diet. Ingredients such as glucomannan, fiber, and Garcinia Cambogia are common in appetite-suppressing supplements. By increasing satiety, these supplements help prevent overeating.

3. THERMOGENICS: These supplements aim to increase your metabolic rate, making your body burn more calories throughout the day. Ingredients like green tea extract, caffeine, and cayenne pepper are common in thermogenic supplements. While effective, they should be used with caution due to their stimulating effects on the nervous system.

4. FAT BLOCKERS: Fat blockers, such as Orlistat, prevent the absorption of dietary fat. These supplements can be useful for individuals who struggle with consuming excess fats in their diet. However, they may cause gastrointestinal issues, so it is crucial to take them as directed.

5. PROTEIN SUPPLEMENTS: Protein is an essential nutrient that can aid weight loss by promoting muscle repair and growth. Whey protein, casein protein, and plant-based proteins (like pea or hemp protein) are popular choices. Protein supplements can help reduce hunger and increase your metabolism, especially when consumed after a workout.

84.3 IMPORTANT CONSIDERATIONS BEFORE USING WEIGHT LOSS SUPPLEMENTS

Before diving into the world of weight loss supplements, it's important to keep these considerations in mind:

1. CONSULT A HEALTHCARE PROFESSIONAL: Some weight loss supplements may interact with medications or have adverse effects for people with certain health conditions. It's always wise to consult a doctor or nutritionist before starting any supplement, especially if you have existing health issues or are taking medication.

2. READ THE LABEL: Many weight loss supplements contain hidden ingredients or excessive amounts of stimulants that can cause unwanted side effects such as jitteriness, anxiety, or digestive issues. Always read the label thoroughly and be cautious of any "miracle" claims.

3. AVOID EXCESSIVE DOSING: Some individuals believe that taking more than the recommended dose will speed up weight loss, but this is not the case. Taking excessive amounts of supplements can lead to side effects and even serious health issues. Stick to the recommended dosage and avoid combining multiple supplements that have overlapping ingredients.

4. NATURAL vs. SYNTHETIC: There is a difference between natural supplements (like those derived from plants) and synthetic ones. Natural supplements often come with fewer side effects, but they may be less potent than their synthetic counterparts. Choose based on your body's response and preference.

84.4 EFFECTIVE WEIGHT LOSS SUPPLEMENTS AND THEIR BENEFITS

Here are a few weight loss supplements with proven effectiveness:

1. GREEN TEA EXTRACT: Green tea extract is rich in antioxidants known as catechins. These compounds help to increase fat oxidation, especially during exercise. Green tea also contains a small amount of caffeine, which can improve energy levels and help burn fat.

2. GARCINIA CAMBOGIA: This tropical fruit extract contains hydroxycitric acid (HCA), which is believed to reduce appetite and prevent fat storage. Studies suggest that it can assist with weight loss by inhibiting the enzyme that converts carbohydrates into fat.

3. CAFFEINE: A well-known stimulant, caffeine boosts metabolism and increases fat burning, especially during exercise. It also helps improve focus and energy, which can aid in sticking to a workout routine. However, it should be used in moderation to avoid the negative side effects of excess stimulation.

4. CLA (CONJUGATED LINOLEIC ACID): CLA is a naturally occurring fatty acid found in meat and dairy products. Some studies suggest that CLA can help reduce body fat by increasing the rate at which your body burns fat. It also has muscle-preserving benefits, which is important when you're in a calorie deficit.

5. FIBER SUPPLEMENTS: Soluble fiber supplements, such as psyllium husk, can help curb hunger by promoting feelings of fullness. Fiber also supports digestive health and may aid in fat absorption, making it easier for your body to process food efficiently.

84.5 CONCLUSION: USING SUPPLEMENTS TO SUPPORT A WELL-ROUNDED WEIGHT LOSS PLAN

Weight loss supplements can be an effective addition to a healthy weight loss strategy when used properly. However, they should never replace the foundation of healthy eating and regular exercise. Supplements work best when they complement a balanced diet, sufficient sleep, stress management, and consistent physical activity. Always choose supplements that align with your specific health needs and consult a healthcare professional before beginning a new regimen. By choosing the right supplements, you can enhance your efforts, support your metabolism, and make your weight loss journey a little easier and more effective.

CHAPTER 85: AVOID ARTIFICIAL SWEETENERS

85.1 UNDERSTANDING ARTIFICIAL SWEETENERS

Artificial sweeteners are synthetic sugar substitutes found in many "sugar-free" or "diet" products, including beverages, desserts, and processed foods. They are designed to provide sweetness without the calories of sugar. Common types include aspartame, sucralose, saccharin, and acesulfame potassium.

While they may seem like a healthier option, artificial sweeteners can pose various health risks and may not support your weight loss goals as effectively as you might think.

85.2 RISKS OF ARTIFICIAL SWEETENERS

1. DISRUPTION OF METABOLISM:
Studies suggest that artificial sweeteners may interfere with the body's ability to regulate glucose, potentially leading to insulin resistance and increased fat storage. This can hinder weight loss efforts and even contribute to weight gain over time.

2. INCREASED SUGAR CRAVINGS:
Ironically, consuming artificial sweeteners can trigger cravings for sugary foods. They may condition your taste buds to expect more sweetness, causing you to seek out high-calorie, sugar-laden treats.

3. POTENTIAL HEALTH CONCERNS:
Long-term use of artificial sweeteners has been linked to various health issues, including headaches, digestive problems, and an increased risk of developing certain chronic diseases. Though more research is needed, some studies also suggest potential links to increased risks of heart disease and certain cancers.

85.3 WHY YOU SHOULD AVOID ARTIFICIAL SWEETENERS

1. FALSE SENSE OF SECURITY:
Artificial sweeteners may make you feel like you're making healthier choices, but they don't necessarily lead to better health outcomes. Relying on these substitutes can lead to overconsumption of other unhealthy foods, negating their calorie-saving benefits.

2. INTERFERENCE WITH GUT HEALTH:
Emerging research indicates that artificial sweeteners can negatively affect gut bacteria, which play a crucial role in digestion, immunity, and overall health. An imbalanced gut microbiome can lead to bloating, poor digestion, and even weight gain.

85.4 HEALTHIER ALTERNATIVES TO ARTIFICIAL SWEETENERS

Instead of artificial sweeteners, consider these natural, healthier options to satisfy your sweet tooth without compromising your health:

1. STEVIA:
Derived from the leaves of the Stevia plant, this natural sweetener contains no calories and has minimal impact on blood sugar levels.

2. MONK FRUIT EXTRACT:
This natural sweetener is derived from monk fruit and offers a calorie-free way to add sweetness to your foods and beverages.

3. HONEY AND MAPLE SYRUP:
Though these contain calories, they are more natural and provide additional nutrients like antioxidants and minerals. Use them sparingly to add flavor without excessive sugar.

85.5 TIPS TO REDUCE YOUR SWEETENERS INTAKE

1. RE-TRAIN YOUR TASTE BUDS:
Gradually reduce your dependence on sweet flavors. Over time, your taste buds will adjust, and you'll find satisfaction in less sweet foods.

2. OPT FOR WHOLE FOODS:
Choose naturally sweet whole foods like fruits to satisfy your cravings. They provide fiber and essential nutrients, making them a healthier alternative.

3. READ LABELS CAREFULLY:
Artificial sweeteners can be hidden in many processed foods. Always check the ingredient list and avoid products with artificial sweeteners.

85.6 THE IMPACT OF AVOIDING ARTIFICIAL SWEETENERS

Eliminating artificial sweeteners from your diet can lead to numerous benefits:

1. BETTER METABOLIC HEALTH:
You'll likely experience improved insulin sensitivity and a more stable blood sugar level, aiding in effective weight management.

2. REDUCED CRAVINGS:
By avoiding artificial sweeteners, you can break the cycle of sugar cravings, making it easier to stick to a healthy eating plan.

3. ENHANCED GUT HEALTH:
A healthier gut microbiome contributes to better digestion, improved immunity, and overall well-being.

4. MORE MINDFUL EATING:
Choosing natural alternatives encourages a more mindful approach to sweetening your foods, promoting healthier eating habits.

85.7 CONCLUSION

While artificial sweeteners are marketed as a healthier alternative to sugar, their long-term effects can undermine your weight loss goals and overall health. By avoiding them and choosing natural alternatives, you can improve your diet, reduce sugar cravings, and enhance your overall well-being. Embrace the change for a healthier lifestyle that prioritizes natural sweetness and balanced nutrition.

CHAPTER 86: TRACK YOUR PROGRESS

86.1 WHY TRACKING IS IMPORTANT

Tracking your weight loss progress allows you to see how far you've come and can help you stay motivated. Regular tracking also helps identify areas for improvement and ensures you're staying on track with your goals. Monitoring your progress gives you a clear picture of what works and allows for adjustments to your diet and exercise plan.

86.2 WAYS TO TRACK PROGRESS

You can track progress in several ways:

*WEIGHT AND MEASUREMENTS: Weigh yourself weekly and take body measurements (waist, hips, chest, etc.) to track changes in body composition.

*PROGRESS PHOTOS: Take photos every few weeks to visually assess changes.

*FITNESS PROGRESS: Track your workouts, including improvements in strength, stamina, or flexibility.

*FOOD JOURNAL: Keep track of your meals and snacks to understand your eating habits better.

86.3 AVOID OBSESSING OVER THE SCALE

While tracking weight is important, it's essential not to obsess over the scale. Weight fluctuations are normal due to factors like water retention and muscle gain. Focus on overall progress rather than just the numbers on the scale.

CHAPTER 87: CREATE A SUPPORT SYSTEM

87.1 WHY A SUPPORT SYSTEM MATTERS

Having a support system is essential for staying motivated and accountable throughout your weight loss journey. Whether it's friends, family, or online communities, sharing your goals and challenges with others can help keep you on track. Support systems provide emotional encouragement, accountability, and practical advice.

87.2 HOW TO BUILD A SUPPORT SYSTEM

Join a weight loss group or find a workout buddy to help motivate you. Engage with others who share similar goals and offer mutual support. Be open with your close friends and family about your goals, so they can provide encouragement and help keep you accountable.

87.3 ONLINE COMMUNITIES AND RESOURCES

There are plenty of online forums, apps, and social media groups where you can connect with others working on weight loss. Consider joining platforms like MyFitnessPal, Reddit's weight loss communities, or Facebook groups dedicated to health and fitness.

CHAPTER 88: EAT MORE WHOLE FOODS

88.1 WHAT ARE WHOLE FOODS?

Whole foods are foods that are minimally processed and free from additives and preservatives. These foods include fruits, vegetables, whole grains, nuts, seeds, and lean proteins. They are rich in nutrients, vitamins, minerals, and fiber, which are essential for maintaining good health and supporting weight loss.

88.2 BENEFITS OF EATING WHOLE FOODS

Eating whole foods is beneficial because they provide more fiber and fewer empty calories than processed foods. Fiber helps you feel full, which can prevent overeating. Whole foods are also packed with antioxidants, which reduce inflammation and improve overall health. These foods help stabilize blood sugar levels, reduce cravings, and promote fat loss.

88.3 HOW TO INCORPORATE MORE WHOLE FOODS INTO YOUR DIET

To increase your intake of whole foods, start by filling your plate with vegetables, fruits, and whole grains. Choose lean meats and fish over processed meats, and swap refined grains for whole grains like brown rice, quinoa, and whole wheat bread. Make sure that every meal includes a good portion of whole foods.

CHAPTER 89: USE HEALTHY SUBSTITUTES FOR BAKING

89.1 THE NEED FOR HEALTHIER BAKING

Traditional baking often relies on ingredients like refined sugar, white flour, and butter, which can be high in calories and low in nutrients. While these staples provide flavor and texture, they may not align with health-conscious eating or weight loss goals. Fortunately, healthier substitutes can offer similar results with added nutritional benefits.

Incorporating healthy alternatives into your baking not only supports your dietary goals but also enhances the nutritional profile of your baked goods.

89.2 COMMON HEALTHY BAKING SUBSTITUTES

1. REPLACING SUGAR:
Refined sugar is a major contributor to empty calories. Consider the following alternatives:

*HONEY OR MAPLE SYRUP: These natural sweeteners provide sweetness with added nutrients like antioxidants and minerals.

*STEVIA OR MONK FRUIT EXTRACT: These zero-calorie sweeteners are plant-based and have minimal impact on blood sugar levels.

*MASHED BANANAS OR APPLESAUCE: Both offer natural sweetness along with fiber and vitamins.

2. REPLACING BUTTER:
Butter adds flavor but is high in saturated fat. Healthier options include:

*COCONUT OIL: A plant-based fat that offers a mild sweetness. Use it in moderation.

*GREEK YOGURT: Provides creaminess while reducing fat content and adding protein.

*MASHED AVOCADO: A nutrient-dense alternative that works well in recipes like brownies or muffins.

3. REPLACING WHITE FLOUR:
White flour lacks fiber and nutrients. Opt for:

*WHOLE WHEAT FLOUR: Contains more fiber and nutrients, offering a denser texture.

*ALMOND FLOUR: A gluten-free option rich in protein and healthy fats.

OAT FLOUR: Made by grinding oats, it provides fiber and a mild, nutty flavor.

89.3 BENEFITS OF HEALTHY SUBSTITUTES

1. IMPROVED NUTRITIONAL VALUE:
Healthy substitutes increase the fiber, protein, and essential nutrients in your baked goods, making them more filling and beneficial.

2. LOWER CALORIE CONTENT:
By swapping high-calorie ingredients like sugar and butter, you can enjoy your treats without consuming excess calories.

3. BETTER BLOOD SUGAR CONTROL:
Natural sweeteners and whole grains cause slower blood sugar spikes, helping to maintain energy levels and reduce cravings.

4. ACCOMMODATION FOR DIETARY NEEDS:
Using substitutes like almond flour or coconut oil caters to gluten-free, lactose-free, or vegan diets, making your baking more inclusive.

89.4 TIPS FOR USING HEALTHY SUBSTITUTES

1. START SMALL:
When experimenting with substitutes, start by replacing a portion of the original ingredient. For instance, replace half the white flour with almond flour to see how it affects the texture and taste.

2. ADJUST LIQUIDS:
Some substitutes, like applesauce or Greek yogurt, add moisture. You may need to reduce other liquids in the recipe.

3. PAY ATTENTION TO TEXTURE:
Healthy substitutes can alter the texture of baked goods. Whole wheat flour, for example, makes for denser products, while almond flour creates a softer crumb.

4. BALANCE FLAVORS:
Substitutes like mashed avocado or coconut oil have distinct flavors. Pair them with complementary ingredients to maintain the desired taste.

89.5 POPULAR RECIPES WITH HEALTHY SUBSTITUTES

1. WHOLE WHEAT BANANA BREAD:
Swap white flour for whole wheat flour and use mashed bananas as a natural sweetener. Add a touch of honey for extra sweetness.

2. ALMOND FLOUR BROWNIES:
Replace regular flour with almond flour and use unsweetened applesauce instead of butter. Sweeten with monk fruit extract.

3. GREEK YOGURT MUFFINS:
Use Greek yogurt in place of butter for added protein and moisture. Replace half the sugar with honey for a naturally sweetened treat.

89.6 CONCLUSION

Baking with healthy substitutes allows you to enjoy your favorite treats while aligning with your health goals. By incorporating nutrient-rich ingredients, you can create baked goods that are not only delicious but also beneficial for your well-being. With a little experimentation, healthier baking can become a rewarding and enjoyable part of your lifestyle.

CHAPTER 90: STAY POSITIVE THROUGHOUT YOUR JOURNEY

90.1 THE POWER OF A POSITIVE MINDSET

A positive mindset is essential for long-term weight loss success. Focusing on the progress you've made rather than setbacks helps build resilience. A positive attitude can also help you stay motivated and reduce stress, which in turn supports your weight loss efforts.

90.2 STRATEGIES TO MAINTAIN A POSITIVE ATTITUDE

Celebrate small victories along the way, such as reaching a fitness milestone or making healthier food choices. Keep a journal to reflect on your achievements, and surround yourself with positive influences. Avoid negative self-talk, and instead focus on how far you've come and the healthy habits you're building.

90.3 BE KIND TO YOURSELF

Weight loss is a journey with ups and downs. If you slip up, don't be too hard on yourself. Instead of focusing on mistakes, refocus on your goals and move forward with a renewed sense of determination. Self-compassion is key to maintaining motivation and resilience.

CHAPTER 91: AVOID FAD DIETS

91.1 WHY FAD DIETS DON'T WORK

Fad diets promise quick results, but they are often unsustainable and can lead to weight gain once you return to regular eating habits. These diets often restrict essential nutrients and are not based on balanced, long-term healthy eating principles. The rapid weight loss associated with fad diets is often temporary.

91.2 HOW TO SPOT A FAD DIET

Fad diets usually promise dramatic results in a short time and require cutting out entire food groups or eating only one type of food. They often lack scientific evidence and promote unhealthy behaviors, such as extreme calorie restriction or detox cleanses.

91.3 FOCUS ON SUSTAINABLE LIFESTYLE CHANGES

Instead of jumping on the latest diet trend, focus on adopting a balanced, sustainable approach to eating. Incorporate whole, nutritious foods, practice portion control, and stay active. These changes will lead to lasting results without the need for restrictive diets.

CHAPTER 92: FOCUS ON LONG-TERM HEALTH

92.1 WHY LONG-TERM HEALTH MATTERS MORE THAN QUICK FIXES

Quick fixes and rapid weight loss methods may offer immediate results, but they often don't support long-term health. Healthy weight management is about making gradual changes to your lifestyle that you can maintain over time. Focus on developing habits that support your overall well-being, including a balanced diet, regular exercise, and mental health practices.

92.2 THE BENEFITS OF LONG-TERM HEALTH GOALS

Focusing on long-term health promotes sustainable weight loss, improves mental and physical health, and reduces the risk of chronic diseases such as diabetes, heart disease, and high blood pressure. It also helps you feel better, both physically and emotionally.

92.3 HOW TO SET LONG-TERM GOALS

Set realistic, achievable health goals and break them down into smaller steps. Track your progress and make adjustments as needed. Prioritize health over the scale, and focus on building healthy habits that you can maintain for life.

CHAPTER 93: ENJOY YOUR WEIGHT LOSS JOURNEY

93.1 MAKING THE JOURNEY PLEASURABLE

Losing weight is not only about shedding pounds, it's about creating a lifestyle that you enjoy. By making the process fun and rewarding, you're more likely to stay committed. Find exercises, activities, and foods that bring you joy, and incorporate them into your routine. Whether it's dancing, hiking, or cooking healthy meals you love, making these things part of your weight loss journey ensures consistency and long-term success.

93.2 FOCUS ON NON-SCALE VICTORIES

Celebrate victories that go beyond just the number on the scale. Perhaps you notice that you have more energy, your clothes fit better, or you're sleeping more soundly. These non-scale victories can be just as rewarding and will keep you motivated on your journey.

93.3 BE PATIENT WITH YOURSELF

Progress takes time. Be patient and kind to yourself during this journey. It's not about perfection but consistent effort. Focus on your progress, not just your setbacks, and embrace the process as a way to improve your overall well-being.

CHAPTER 94: INCLUDE AVOCADOS IN YOUR DIET

94.1 THE BENEFITS OF AVOCADOS

Avocados are often hailed as a superfood due to their impressive nutritional profile. Packed with healthy fats, fiber, and essential nutrients, they are a versatile addition to any diet. Unlike most fruits, avocados are low in sugar and rich in monounsaturated fats, making them an excellent choice for heart health and weight management.

Adding avocados to your diet can enhance your overall health and support your weight loss goals.

94.2 NUTRIENTS FOUND IN AVOCADOS

1. HEALTHY FATS:
Avocados are rich in monounsaturated fats, which help lower bad cholesterol (LDL) levels while increasing good cholesterol (HDL). These fats provide sustained energy and help you feel full longer.

2. FIBER:
A single avocado contains about 10 grams of fiber, which aids in digestion and promotes a feeling of fullness. Fiber also helps regulate blood sugar levels, reducing spikes and crashes.

3. VITAMINS AND MINERALS:
Avocados are an excellent source of essential vitamins and minerals, including:

*VITAMIN K: Important for blood clotting and bone health.

*VITAMIN E: A powerful antioxidant that protects cells from damage.

*POTASSIUM: Helps regulate blood pressure and supports muscle function.

94.3 HEALTH BENEFITS OF AVOCADOS

1. WEIGHT MANAGEMENT:

The combination of healthy fats and fiber in avocados helps control hunger by keeping you full for longer periods. This reduces the likelihood of overeating and snacking on unhealthy foods.

2. HEART HEALTH:

Avocados support cardiovascular health by lowering cholesterol and triglyceride levels. They also contain potassium, which helps maintain healthy blood pressure.

3. IMPROVED DIGESTION:

The high fiber content promotes healthy digestion and regular bowel movements, preventing constipation and supporting gut health.

4. SKIN AND HAIR HEALTH:

Avocados are rich in antioxidants and healthy fats that nourish the skin and hair, keeping them hydrated and reducing signs of aging.

94.4 HOW TO INCLUDE AVOCADOS IN YOUR DIET

1. BREAKFAST:

*AVOCADO TOAST: Spread mashed avocado on whole-grain toast and top with a pinch of salt, pepper, or a poached egg.

*SMOOTHIES: Blend avocado with spinach, banana, and almond milk for a creamy, nutrient-packed drink.

2. LUNCH AND DINNER:

*SALADS: Add sliced or diced avocado to salads for a boost of healthy fats and creaminess.

*WRAPS AND SANDWICHES: Use avocado as a spread instead of mayonnaise for a healthier alternative.

3. SNACKS:

*GUACAMOLE: Mix mashed avocado with lime juice, garlic, and diced tomatoes for a flavorful dip. Pair it with vegetable sticks or whole-grain chips.

*AVOCADO SLICES: Simply sprinkle with salt and enjoy as a quick snack.

4. DESSERTS:

*AVOCADO CHOCOLATE PUDDING: Blend ripe avocado with cocoa powder, honey, and a splash of almond milk for a rich, healthy dessert.

94.5 TIPS FOR CHOOSING AND STORING AVOCADOS

1. CHOOSING RIPE AVOCADOS:
A ripe avocado yields to gentle pressure without feeling mushy. If it's too firm, leave it at room temperature to ripen over a few days.

2. STORING AVOCADOS:
Once ripe, avocados can be stored in the refrigerator to slow the ripening process. To store a cut avocado, sprinkle it with lemon juice and wrap it tightly in plastic wrap to prevent browning.

94.6 CONCLUSION

Including avocados in your diet is a simple and delicious way to boost your intake of healthy fats, fiber, and essential nutrients. Whether you enjoy them in salads, as a spread, or in smoothies, avocados can support your weight loss journey and overall health. With their versatility and numerous health benefits, avocados deserve a place in your daily meals.

CHAPTER 95: SETTING REALISTIC EXPECTATIONS

95.1 WHY SETTING REALISTIC EXPECTATIONS MATTERS

Setting realistic expectations for your weight loss journey helps prevent frustration and burnout. Unrealistic goals can lead to disappointment, making it harder to stay motivated. When you set achievable goals, you can focus on making steady progress, which is much more sustainable in the long run.

95.2 HOW TO SET REALISTIC WEIGHT LOSS GOALS

Start with small, manageable goals and gradually work up to larger ones. A realistic target is to aim for 1-2 pounds of weight loss per week. Focus on creating habits that you can maintain long-term, rather than quick fixes that are unsustainable. Use specific, measurable, achievable, relevant, and time-bound (SMART) goals to stay on track.

95.3 THE IMPORTANCE OF FLEXIBILITY

Be flexible with your goals and willing to adjust them as needed. Life circumstances may change, and it's important to be adaptable. If you encounter challenges, don't give up. Instead, reevaluate and find new strategies to continue your journey toward a healthier lifestyle.

CHAPTER 96: AVOID THE "ALL OR NOTHING" MINDSET

96.1 THE DANGER OF THE "ALL OR NOTHING" MINDSET

The "all or nothing" mentality can be a major obstacle to long-term success. Thinking that you must follow your weight loss plan perfectly or it's not worth doing at all can lead to feelings of failure and discourage you from continuing. Instead, focus on making progress, even if it's imperfect.

96.2 WHY SMALL CHANGES MATTER

Small, consistent changes add up over time and can lead to significant results. Missing a workout or eating an unhealthy meal doesn't mean you've failed—it's just a minor setback. Focus on getting back on track and continue to build healthy habits that you can maintain long-term.

96.3 HOW TO BREAK FREE FROM ALL-OR-NOTHING THINKING

Challenge the belief that you must be perfect to be successful. Embrace flexibility and focus on making positive choices more often than not. Remember that consistency is more important than perfection. Celebrate small wins and forgive yourself when things don't go as planned.

CHAPTER 97: INCORPORATE REGULAR PHYSICAL ACTIVITY

97.1 THE ROLE OF EXERCISE IN WEIGHT LOSS

Exercise is essential for weight loss and overall health. It helps burn calories, increases metabolism, improves cardiovascular health, and enhances mood. A combination of aerobic exercises, strength training, and flexibility exercises is ideal for maximizing fat loss and building muscle.

97.2 HOW MUCH EXERCISE IS ENOUGH?

Aim for at least 150 minutes of moderate-intensity exercise per week, or 75 minutes of vigorous-intensity exercise, along with two or more days of strength training. You can break this up into smaller sessions throughout the week to make it more manageable.

97.3 FINDING AN EXERCISE ROUTINE YOU ENJOY

The key to consistency in exercise is enjoying what you do. Whether it's walking, cycling, swimming, or group fitness classes, find activities that you look forward to. This will make it easier to stick to your workout plan and make exercise a permanent part of your lifestyle.

CHAPTER 98: REWARD YOURSELF

98.1 THE IMPORTANCE OF REWARDS

Rewarding yourself for reaching milestones keeps you motivated and reinforces your healthy habits. However, it's essential to choose rewards that are not food-related, as food rewards can hinder your progress. Instead, focus on rewards that promote well-being or further your goals.

98.2 NON-FOOD REWARDS IDEAS

Consider treating yourself to a relaxing spa day, a new workout outfit, or a fun activity like a movie night or a weekend getaway. You can also reward yourself with new fitness equipment or a personal fitness tracker to track your progress.

98.3 THE POWER OF SMALL REWARDS

Small rewards along the way can make your weight loss journey more enjoyable. After achieving small goals, reward yourself with things that make you feel good and encourage you to keep going.

CHAPTER 99: STAY COMMITTED THROUGH CHALLENGES

99.1 EXPECTING CHALLENGES ON THE JOURNEY

Weight loss is rarely a smooth path. You will face obstacles, setbacks, and challenges. Understanding that these are part of the journey can help you stay committed. The key is not to let challenges derail your progress but to use them as opportunities for growth.

99.2 OVERCOMING OBSTACLES

When faced with challenges, take a step back and assess the situation. Ask yourself what went wrong, and what you can learn from it. Plan ahead for potential challenges and prepare strategies to stay on track. Having a support system in place can also help you stay motivated during tough times.

99.3 STAYING FOCUSED ON YOUR GOALS

Keep your long-term goals in mind, and don't let temporary setbacks deter you. Every small step forward, no matter how insignificant it may seem, is a step closer to your goal. Stay focused on the big picture, and don't let short-term struggles define your progress.

CHAPTER 100: MAINTAINING YOUR WEIGHT LOSS

100.1 THE IMPORTANCE OF MAINTENANCE

Once you've reached your weight loss goal, maintaining that weight is a new challenge. It's essential to continue healthy habits to prevent regaining the weight. Maintenance requires ongoing effort, including a balanced diet, regular physical activity, and mindfulness about your food choices.

100.2 HOW TO MAINTAIN YOUR RESULTS

To maintain your weight loss, continue the habits that got you there. This includes eating a balanced diet, exercising regularly, and staying mindful of your portion sizes. Be consistent with your healthy habits, but allow yourself flexibility to enjoy life and occasional treats.

100.3 BE PREPARED FOR LIFE CHANGES

Life events such as holidays, vacations, or stressful times can impact your ability to stay on track. Prepare for these situations by planning ahead and making adjustments to your routine when needed. Stay focused on long-term health and wellness, and remember that a temporary slip-up doesn't mean failure.

CONCLUSION:

Achieving and maintaining a healthy weight is a journey that requires dedication, consistency, and informed decision-making. The 100 tips outlined in this book serve as a comprehensive guide to help you navigate the challenges of weight loss and embrace a healthier lifestyle.

Weight loss is not a one-size-fits-all process. It involves a combination of healthy eating, regular physical activity, mindful habits, and lifestyle adjustments tailored to your individual needs. From setting realistic goals and tracking your progress to incorporating more nutrient-dense foods and staying hydrated, each tip plays a crucial role in creating sustainable change.

Moreover, addressing mental and emotional well-being is equally important. Managing stress, practicing self-discipline, and building a support system contribute significantly to long-term success. Remember, setbacks are a natural part of the journey. Instead of dwelling on them, use them as learning experiences to strengthen your resolve.

Ultimately, the path to weight loss is about more than just shedding pounds. It's about building a healthier, more vibrant you. By applying the insights and strategies provided in this book, you can create a balanced lifestyle that not only helps you reach your weight loss goals but also enhances your overall well-being for years to come.

www.ingramcontent.com/pod-product-compliance
Lightning Source LLC
Chambersburg PA
CBHW081220260726
48653CB00010BB/3721